Xandria Williams began her career as a geo........ involved in mineral exploration but soon turned to biochemistry and the study of nutrition, naturopathy, homeopathy and botanic medicine. She then extended her studies to Neurolinguistic Programming, Time-Line Therapy, Voice Dialogue and many other methods of helping people with emotional, personal and psychological problems.

She has lectured extensively at many natural therapies colleges and conferences and holds classes and seminars on a range of aspects of physical, mental and emotional health care. She has written several hundred articles, has often been heard on radio and television and is the author of *Living with Allergies*, *What's in your Food*, *Osteoporosis*, *Choosing Health Intentionally*, *Choosing Weight Intentionally*, *Stress – Recognise and Resolve*, *Beating the Blues*, *Love Health & Happiness* and *Liver Detox Plan*.

Xandria Williams has evolved her unique and highly effective approach to tackling life's problems over two decades of research into helping people at her clinics, in her seminars and through her books and articles.

Xandria is currently in practice in central London and can be contacted for consultations.

28 Lower Sloane Street, London SW1W 8BJ
Phone/fax 0171 824 8153, Email xkw@bigfoot.com

XANDRIA WILLIAMS

Fatigue

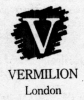

VERMILION
London

1 3 5 7 9 10 8 6 4 2

First published by Cedar in 1996.
This edition published in 2000 by Vermilion,
an imprint of Ebury Press, Random House,
20 Vauxhall Bridge Road, London SW1V 2SA
www.randomhouse.co.uk

Random House Australia (Pty) Limited
20 Alfred Street, Milsons Point, Sydney,
New South Wales 2061, Australia

Random House New Zealand Limited
18 Poland Road, Glenfield,
Auckland 10, New Zealand

Random House South Africa (Pty) Limited
Endulini, 5A Jubilee Road,
Parktown 2193, South Africa

The Random House Group Limited Reg No. 954009

Papers used by Vermilion are natural, recyclable products
made from wood grown in sustainable forests.

Printed and bound by Bookcraft, Bath

A CIP catalogue record for this book
is available from the British Library

ISBN 0-7493-2066-4

Contents

Introduction

Taking Energy for Granted

It is easy to take energy for granted ... until something goes wrong. As a young person, you expect to bounce out of bed, to be able to walk, run, play, and do all the things you want. At the end of an active day, it comes as no surprise that you are tired and want to rest, but you do so sure in the knowledge that you will soon, after the appropriate rest, bounce back and be full of energy once again. This casual assumption of energy usually continues into the teens and, if you are lucky, beyond. Most people expect to have plenty of energy until they reach what they consider to be the apex of their life and then to have diminishing energy which they will attribute to the passing years and the approach of old age.

Sadly, events may overtake you. You may run out of energy prematurely. You may find, even if you are in your thirties, your twenties, possibly even in your teens or a child, that your energy is gradually diminishing, you need more rest than before, and cannot do as much as you once did. You may even find that the energy you once relied upon is suddenly no longer there. It may have dropped after a pregnancy, an illness, or a particularly stressful period. Or it may have lapsed for no apparent reason.

Many patients have expressed surprise when complaining of fatigue; but there is nothing strange about it. It's a bit like an inheritance: you can live high on the hog while it lasts, but when it runs out the question 'I've always spent this much, why can I no longer do so?' has an obvious answer – your money has run out, your expenditure has been greater than your income and you are now broke. In energy terms, the situation is similar. You were born with certain assets. You have now used up your nutritional inheritance. Your nutritional input has been insufficient to keep up with your expenditure or requirements. Your account is exhausted, and so are you.

Putting the situation right may simply entail increasing your 'income' by raising your nutritional input, improving the quality of your diet, or taking supplements. It may mean correcting some relatively minor health problem such as hypoglycaemia, allergies or anaemia. Alternatively, it may mean correcting a more severe health problem such as a heart problem or an endocrine imbalance. Exhaustion that is not relieved by any of these relatively simple means may prove to be full-blown Chronic Fatigue Syndrome (CFS). This is a more serious situation and may take longer to correct.

In this book, we shall be covering fatigue at all these levels. The good news is that in virtually every case, whether the fatigue is (relatively) simple or chronic, positive results are possible. The less good news is that it may take more time and more effort than you thought or would like. But persevere. Getting your energy back is important, possible and well worth the effort.

Energy

Do you have all the energy you need? Probably not, or you wouldn't have picked this book up. Are you trying to do too much? You may think so, and indeed this may be true. But are you only trying to do too much in terms of the amount of energy you have? Do you feel you are short of energy rather than long on things to do? Quite probably. Do you look around and see other people with more energy than you, people who can skip through the day coping with all that is asked of them, who feel pleasantly tired at the end of the day, satisfied with what they have accomplished and content to relax and unwind, whereas you slump exhausted into a chair, too tired to enjoy even the little bit of spare time you have?

The majority of my patients complain of being tired. It may be that tiredness is their prime presenting symptom, it may be one of several problems that they have come to tell me about, or it may be a symptom that accompanies the main problem that has brought them in, something they mention only as an afterthought. However the information is offered, it becomes part of the equation, part of the information that provides clues and that, ultimately, is used to formulate the treatment.

Other patients may fail to recognise their lowered energy level, or not think it worth mentioning or that anything can be done about it. They present a set of symptoms, are helped with these problems and then, at the end of the treatment, they report that not only has their presenting problem gone but at the same time their energy has increased.

Still others may never have experienced vibrant energy. I recall one friend who assured me she was fit and well, full of energy and had no health problems whatsoever. She was already taking a multivitamin and a multimineral supplement each day and claimed to need nothing more. I offered her a challenge. She was to take the same supplement programme that I was taking – which I, obviously, considered was the best! – and see how she felt. Within a month she phoned me to say she had never felt better in her life and that she 'hadn't realised you could feel this good'. It is sad to think how many lives are lived in a state of unrecognised tiredness; a tiredness that the person takes for granted yet could so easily be changed.

There are all sorts of patterns of energy and of fatigue. You may find you feel full of beans in the morning, but are exhausted by the end of the day and have just enough energy to eat a meal and slouch in front of the television. Other people find that there are particular times of the day when they feel tired. For some, this is the afternoon slump. For others, exhaustion strikes mid-morning. Some feel revived after an hour or two, others may feel tired for the rest of the day.

Then again, there are the night owls. Maybe getting out of bed is a struggle. Getting started is difficult and your friends and colleagues know not to talk to you till lunch-time. You have little energy during the day but come awake during the evening, and stay up late, the life and soul of the party, able to concentrate and create, love and play, with all the energy that was conspicuously lacking in the morning. Wouldn't it be nice to have that sort of energy all day long?

In the most debilitated category are those suffering from chronic fatigue. They wake up tired and drag themselves through the day, never having the energy to do anything easily, not getting their tasks done, possibly not even able to work or run the home. They spend a lot of the day resting and then collapse into bed in the middle of the evening. This may simply be a generalised low energy level or it might be full-blown Chronic

Fatigue Syndrome with its accompanying symptoms such as joint and limb pain, headaches and more.

Energy is such a fundamental requirement that you should be seriously concerned when the amount you have available proves inadequate, not only when the problem is obviously serious, as in Chronic Fatigue Syndrome, but even when your level is only slightly below normal. Without energy, you cannot function. No matter how wonderful your car, without petrol it won't run. No matter how fantastic your high-tech equipment, without electricity it is useless. No matter how good your ideas and intentions, without energy you cannot put them into practice. You too need the proper fuel input and proper maintenance.

There is another very important point. It is not simply a question of whether or not you have enough energy to get by. A low level of energy production means more than the simple fact that you are tired. It also indicates that there are serious problems in the body. They may be simple, such as minor vitamin deficiencies and tired adrenal glands; or they could be major, such as serious hormonal problems, problems related to your heart and lungs, thrush, allergies, diabetes, or cancer. In other words, tiredness is a problem in itself. It is also a symptom, a warning that something else may be wrong. If you feel tired, now is the time to investigate and to fix the problem. Prevention is better than cure and as soon as you don't have all the energy you need and want, that is the moment to start doing something about it.

There are two broad approaches we shall be taking to fatigue and lack of energy in this book. Firstly, there is the general lack of energy, associated with doing too much, insufficient nourishment, becoming run down, or the existence of other health problems. These will be covered in Parts I, II and III. For want of a better term, we shall call this 'simple fatigue'. Secondly, there is Chronic

Fatigue Syndrome (CFS). CFS is addressed in Part IV. It is not just a more severe case of the tiredness described and discussed in Parts I, II and III, although many people often assume this to be so. None the less, the therapies suggested in Parts I, II and III may help alleviate even severe CFS symptoms. However, as you will discover, there are times when the same rules definitely do not apply to someone suffering from CFS. You may already have tried some of the suggestions from the first three Parts and found they didn't work. This does not mean that they are not valid suggestions for the majority of people experiencing fatigue. It simply means that at your stage of CFS they are either not appropriate for you or there is more that has to be done. Do not give up on the therapy and call it useless, even if it doesn't work for you.

There is a final and important point to make at this stage. Individuals are unique and in your particular situation some variations to the general treatments suggested here may be needed. This is true of both simple fatigue and CFS and you may want to talk with a practitioner to complete the process of full recovery.

PART I

Chapter One

Normal Energy Production

For many people, 'energy' is a nebulous concept. It means being able to do things without getting tired, certainly. You know when you have it, you also know when you don't, but just exactly what it is, how you get it, store it or make it available for use, these are things you may not have thought about in any detail. Now is the time to do so.

If you want energy to power your Walkman so you can listen to a tape, what do you do? You put some batteries in the proper compartment of the machine and switch on. So far so good, but how do the batteries get their energy? Perhaps you have rechargeable batteries. If you do, you will know that you put them into wired-up slots in the charger, connect this to the power point and draw on the town's electricity supply. Fine, but where does this energy come from? It may well come from a power station fuelled by coal or gas. It may also come from nuclear or hydroelectric power sources or even from solar power, but for the purposes of this analogy, we shall focus on the first two, coal and gas.

Your body acts in a similar way. It takes in food (like

the coal or gas of the power station) and burns this up
– oxidises it – to release the stored energy. This energy
then has to be stored; first in large storage depots or
molecules, like the local power grid of your town; and
then in small, high-energy molecules, like the batteries.
These smaller molecules or batteries can then move to
wherever the energy is wanted and release it into the
cells (or into the Walkman). The cells can then function,
as can the Walkman.

We can abbreviate and tabulate this as follows:

Original coal or gas	The food you eat
Power station storage	Triglycerides stored in your adipose tissues, and glycogen
Energy available from the local grid or power point	Glucose and fatty acids travelling through the bloodstream
Recharged batteries, ready to deliver	Small molecules called ATP

Let's look at this in more detail and go through the
steps that are required for you to convert your raw
materials, the foods you eat, the air you breathe and the
fluids you drink, into energy in a form that you can use.

Energy Management and Production

1 Your energy comes from the food, drink and air you
take in.

We shall ignore the pleasurable and social reasons for
eating – you have probably given them sufficient
thought already. We shall be considering the needs of
your body, not those of your taste buds. If we do that,
we can say that, from a physiological point of view, you
eat for two reasons: for matter and energy, for structure
and function. You eat to obtain the substances you need

to maintain the physical substance of your body – the flesh and bones, the blood and organs, the nerves, the glands and the hormones.

It is the second reason that interests us here. The second role of eating is to provide you with the *energy* you need to *function*. You need energy at all levels, as an individual, for your organs, for every single cell in your body and even for the parts of the cells to function. Food on its own is not enough. You need air – preferably clean, fresh air – to provide the oxygen that allows you to burn the foods and convert them into energy. You also need water – again, preferably clean, fresh water – to provide the fluid medium in which all the necessary reactions can happen. Dry cells will not function, nor will dry organs and tissues. Dry mucous membranes will tear and be damaged and if you do not drink enough – preferably two to three litres a day – your kidneys will be compromised.

2 The foods you eat are digested, broken down, in the digestive tract, absorbed and made ready for the first oxidation. (This is like getting the coal ready for the furnace.)

3 Then one of two things happens. Either:
(a) it is broken down completely for the generation of immediate energy as described below, or:
(b) these digested nutrients are rearranged within the cells into either glycogen, made up of glucose units and stored in the muscles and liver or, more commonly, into fatty acids and then triglycerides and sent to the adipose tissues for storage. (Like the town's electricity storage station.)

4 When energy is needed subsequently (i.e. some time after eating), then these stored compounds, the glycogen and triglycerides, are released or broken down and fatty acids and glucose circulate in the bloodstream. (Like the power available at your power point when you switch it on, and that can be drawn on by the battery charger.)

5 When these molecules are taken up by a cell (or battery charger) they are 'burned' within the cells and their energy reduced into smaller and more manageable packages (the molecule ATP in the cell or the batteries for your Walkman). For this process to occur, you need the oxygen you've absorbed from the air you breathe, which is circulating in the red blood cells attached to haemoglobin.

6 Once made, the ATP is available wherever it is needed, just as the recharged battery can be put into any piece of battery-operated electrical equipment. This can be inside or outside the cell; it can be used to set off a particular reaction – building your tissues, activating hormones or triggering a nerve cell's response.

If you are healthy and well fed, this process should work smoothly and efficiently and you should have all the energy you need to do whatever you want, within reason.

If you do not have sufficient energy, then either:

1 You are not eating enough (there is a lack of the proper type of raw fuel materials), or:
2 The fuel was not prepared properly for the power station (poor digestion, absorption and assimilation), or:
3 The process of converting the raw material into energy is not working efficiently (you are lacking the trace nutrients, the vitamins and minerals that 'oil' the mechanism and make sure all the proper energy-producing reactions can happen), or:
4 You are not healthy (the equipment is faulty), or:
5 A combination of these factors is involved.

From this, you can see that there are clear steps along the way that are easily identified. If you do not have sufficient energy, it is possible to establish which steps are faulty and there are actions you can take to increase it, up to the limit of your maximum potential. This is done by improving your nutrition – the quality of the fuel, (fats, proteins and carbohydrates) or the facilitating nutrients (the vitamins and minerals) – or by improving your health, or both.

These steps are described in Parts I and II (generating more energy in a body that is generally healthy but is poorly nourished) and Part III (generating more energy in a body that is not healthy by first improving the health of the body). Part IV deals specifically with Chronic Fatigue Syndrome, a syndrome that requires specialised treatment based on an understanding of the fundamental causes of CFS, causes that go beyond those of 'simple fatigue'. CFS does not respond to an unstructured application of the methods described for energy production in someone who is essentially healthy but tired. As you read about the treatment of CFS you will realise that many, possibly all, of the methods used for treating simple fatigue are appropriate, but that more is needed and that the process has to be a lot more thorough and all-embracing.

Let's go back to our analogy. It is also worth pointing out that:

- Some bodies (like some cassette players) have unusually high energy (nutrient) requirements. If you have unusually high nutrient requirements – either for the quantity of food you need or, more usually, for the type of food and the amount of trace nutrients, vitamins and minerals, that you need – these can be provided once the problem has been

recognised. Provided you continue to give your
body this high level of nutritional intake on a daily
basis, you can continue to have a high level of
energy output.

- Some bodies (also like some cassette players) can
  only achieve a somewhat lower-than-average
  maximum energy output. This too can be improved,
  but this time only up to a point. Beyond that point,
  this factor has to be recognised and taken into
  consideration. There are, for instance, some people
  who, no matter how healthy and well-nourished they
  are, will always have lower maximum energy than
  some of their counterparts.

  If you are, inherently, someone who will never have
  a huge amount of energy, someone who is not a get-
  up-and-go person, but a more relaxed and laid-back
  person, then you may never make the change and
  become a high-energy person, no matter how well you
  nourish yourself. However, it is still possible to help
  you achieve your own maximum energy production
  and optimum health.

  Do not give up before you start. Do not assume you
  are a low-energy person and nothing can be done.
  Explore first and find out, with all the help this book[1]
  can give you, just how much energy and good health
  you actually can have.

These two factors relate to your biochemical individuality, to your genes and the way your body functions.
Just as everyone has their own set of genes, everyone
also has their own maximum energy potential. They also
have their own individual nutrient requirements, both
for energy and for optimum health. It is up to you to
find out what you need to do to have the amount of
energy you want.

If just reading this and realising, for the first time, all the steps involved makes you feel tired, don't despair. Like the king and queen who give no thought to how their food is prepared, how their accounts are kept or how their staff are managed, you need give no thought as to how the details are carried out, any more than you worry about how your car or television work internally. You simply do the basics and then use them. It is the same with your body. What you do have to do is to provide it with all the proper fuel (the coal or gas in our analogy above), all the proper tools, the vitamins and minerals, to enable the correct release, control and management of this energy source, and the proper body (power station) for the full release of this energy, in the form of a well-functioning digestive system and healthy cells.

To a certain extent, this becomes a circular situation. You will be able to release, store and manage your energy properly if you are healthy, and you will be healthy if you provide your body with the proper fuel and nutrients so it can do this. To get more energy, you have to break into that cycle and give it a boost, in whatever way is called for by your particular state of health.

The difference between supplying your car and your television on the one hand and your body on the other is that in the case of your body the issue becomes clouded by your emotional needs, your sense of taste, social issues and the varying opinions of dozens of untrained but enthusiastic amateurs to whom you are willing to listen.

Now it is time for you to learn exactly what it is that your body needs in the way of raw materials and exactly how it should function to produce its maximum energy output. For this reason, you will find that some detailed explanations are given as to how your body works and why it needs what it does. This has been kept as simple as possible so that you can read the book and learn what you need without being overwhelmed with detail. However, I stress again, it seems that the more thoroughly people understand the reasons why they should change their diet, alter their lifestyle, take nutritional supplements and modify their current practices, the more willing they are not only to make the changes but to stick to them. If you find some of the explanations too detailed, skip over them. For some people it is enough to know that the reasons exist, to know that they can turn back the pages and check why the various steps are being recommended.

The Steps Along the Way

To understand many of the steps you will be asked to take to improve your energy levels, it is important for you to know what is needed for the normal production of energy within your body. You will then be more willing to modify your lifestyle and give up some of the things (the bad habits) you currently consider to be important. Some patients are willing to take whatever supplements are prescribed until their health improves, and are then willing to take the appropriate reduced/ maintenance intake. Others listen to the instructions, look slightly glazed, start taking the supplements for a while and then stop. If, on the other hand, these patients have a greater awareness of the steps involved and why the relevant nutrients are needed, they make more serious attempts to increase the nutritional quality of their diet and to take the necessary supplements on a regular basis.

The biggest change often occurs when someone actually sees the state of their cells. We achieve this by looking at a thin drop of blood under the microscope, while the cells are still alive.

> *Genevieve was a typical example. On her first visit, she had argued that she did eat a good diet (but see Chapter Two) and that she didn't need to either change it or take supplements. She would, however, take her homeopathic remedy. On her next visit she said she was still tired and that something more had to be done, yet she still felt she didn't need to take vitamins, she ate well and that all that was required was a different remedy. This time, as planned, we took a look at her blood cells. Once she saw the way they either broke down within seconds or stuck together in clumps, she was more than willing to make the necessary changes. She could see that, structurally and functionally, her cells were not performing correctly. I was able to explain what was needed to repair each aspect that was wrong and she was willing to take the appropriate supplements. In next to no time, she had more energy and, when we next looked at her blood film, it was clear that her cells were strong: they didn't break down and they didn't stick together.*

Foods

For normal energy production, the right food must be chosen, with a full complement of all the necessary macronutrients. This means a diet made up mainly of foods rich in complex carbohydrates and low-fat proteins that includes an adequate supply of the trace nutrients, the vitamins, minerals and other nutritional factors.

We will consider the carbohydrates first. One type of complex carbohydrate is commonly called *fibre*. This is not necessarily fibrous at all, although some of it, such as the strings along the length of a celery stalk, obviously is. A better name for it would be 'non-digestible carbo-hydrate', since its main advantage is that it is not digested or broken down in the mouth, stomach or small intestine, but survives to reach the colon. Here it does two things. Firstly, it combines with water to increase the bulk of the waste material passing along the colon and then out as stools. Secondly, some of it acts as food for the beneficial organisms that you want to have living in that part of your body. It is the water held in the fibre plus the mass of dead organisms that makes up the bulk of the stool, and the softer and bulkier it is, the less likely you are to be constipated.

Another type of complex carbohydrate is *starch*, a glu-cose polymer (a huge molecule made up of thousands of glucose molecules all joined together). Starches are found in grains, legumes and vegetables; in fact, they are the major component of most of these foods, other than water. To a lesser extent, they exist in fruits. Starch acts as an efficient energy source for the body.

Simple carbohydrates are the sugars. These come from some vegetables but mainly from fruits. They include the monosaccharides or single sugars called glucose, fructose and galactose, and the disaccharides or double sugars, such as lactose in milk (made up of glucose and galactose joined in pairs), maltose (made up of two glu-cose units joined in pairs and found in malt), and sucrose (made up of glucose and fructose joined in pairs and found in the sugar bowl and in soft drinks and all the other manufactured sugar-laden foods). You will obtain the simple sugars from milk and fruit and also from the breakdown of the complex starches into maltose. These foods contain lots of additional micronutrients as an added bonus – those all-important vitamins and min-erals. You do not, no matter how much you wish it were otherwise, have any nutritional need for sucrose – the sugar found in the sugar bowl!

Strictly speaking, you do not need the simple sugars from fruit, since you could get them by breaking down starch. However, you will benefit from the vitamins and minerals in fruits, from the fibre (although they often contain relatively little) and from the other nutritive factors such as the bioflavonoids. So enjoy your fruit, including the simple sugars in it.

In addition to the carbohydrates, there should also be sufficient protein in your diet to provide the amino acids necessary for rebuilding and repairing your own muscle (protein) tissues. The best source of this protein is wild fish and wild animals. Once fish or animals are farmed and start to lead a sedentary life, the level of their body fat rises dramatically (just as it does in humans!) and so does its degree of saturation. Thus fish is a better source of low-fat protein than farmed and domesticated animals and poultry, since fish are still swimming wild. This is less true, of course, of 'farmed' fish.

A small amount of fat is also necessary in your diet. You need sufficient to supply the essential fatty acids you need daily. This is no excuse to dip into the cream pot, pour vast amounts of mayonnaise over your salads, sla- ther lashings of butter on your bread or eat fried foods. You only need a small amount of fat a day and it should come from nuts and seeds and foods such as avocados and olives.

There should also be an adequate supply of all the vit- amins, minerals and other micronutrients the body needs. The best source of these is vegetables, followed closely by whole grains, low-fat proteins and fruit – foods we have already seen that you should be eating (see Chapters Six and Seven).

Digestion

The next step is digestion, the breaking down of this
food into its components. Carbohydrates break down
into glucose. The simple sugars into their three components, glucose, fructose and galactose. Later on, as we
shall see, the fructose and galactose are converted into
glucose. Proteins break down into individual amino
acids of which there are approximately twenty that make
up the long protein chains found in food. Fats break
down into fatty acids and glycerol. (Most of the fat you
eat is made up of three fatty acids combined with glycerol, hence the name 'triglycerides'.)

This process starts in the mouth, with thorough chewing. This leads to the physical breakdown of food into
tiny particles more easily attacked by chemical digestive
agents. Chewing also leads to the production of saliva,
which helps to hold the food together and facilitate its
transport, and to the release of enzymes, the biological
catalysts necessary for this chemical breakdown to occur.

When this process is complete, the food passes down
the oesophagus and into the stomach. You should be
relaxed and upright, so there is no regurgitation. Hydrochloric acid is produced from special cells in the stomach
wall. Protein-splitting enzymes are also produced. A lot
of mixing takes place here and some digestion occurs,
though only a very small amount.

The next step occurs in the duodenum. This is the
first part of the small intestine, where bile from the gall
bladder and enzymes and digestive juices from the pancreas pour in and act on the food. All three major food
groups are digested here, and in fact this is where the
majority of the digestion occurs. Starch digestion began
in the mouth but the major part of it is done here as
the larger molecules are broken down to disaccharides.
Protein digestion started in the stomach but the majority

of it is completed here. And this is where the triglycerides are broken down into their component fatty acids and glycerol.

The digestive process is completed on the walls of the small intestine where the disaccharides are reduced to single molecules of glucose. The small molecules that result from all this digestion are now ready to be transported across the walls of the small intestine and so absorbed into the bloodstream on the other side.

It is only after this point that you actually absorb the food and it truly enters your body. Up until now, it has been travelling through a long thin tube that passes through you but is not fully part of you. (Small items, such as pips and seeds, can pass straight through and out the other end. Not until they have passed across the intestine wall are they free to move through the bloodstream, throughout your body and become an integral part of it.) It is here, at the walls of the small intestine, that you also absorb the vitamins, minerals and other essential micronutrients. All these molecules are then transported through the bloodstream and delivered to the cells throughout your body as needed. The raw materials have arrived.

You are now ready to let the fibre and other non-digestible material pass on into the large intestine. At this stage, the mixture of waste material, fluids and organisms is very wet. If it stays that way, you will complain of very runny, liquid diarrhoea. As the waste material moves along the large intestine, water is reabsorbed from it back across the colon walls and into the bloodstream. If too much is absorbed you will complain of constipation, dry, hard stools. It is the job of the non-digestible carbohydrate (fibre) to ensure that just the right amount of water is reabsorbed. You will know this ideal situation has been achieved if you pass a bulky and 'mushy' bowel motion as often as you eat a meal. For most people, this is three or four times a day.

Absorption and Transport

Once the molecules have been absorbed across the intestinal wall, they travel through the bloodstream, circulate round the body and are taken up by the cells that need them, as from a continuous passing smorgasbord. All will be well, provided all the nutrients the cells need are present. However, the cells cannot dictate what nutrients are there: all the individual cells can do is hope that the substances they want are there for the taking. Unfortunately, there is no mechanism by which individual cells can get a message to the brain and tell it which specific nutrients are needed. At best, all the brain can do is decide whether to leave the appetite switch on or turn it off. (We shall return to this 'switch' later in the book.)

There are many factors that have to be correct in this process of absorption, transport and cellular uptake. For many substances – such as the fats, vitamin A, iron and copper – specific transport molecules are required. These must be correctly manufactured within the body and be available as needed.

There are receptor sites on the cell walls that make it possible for the cells to take up certain nutrients. These must be active and competent. There are also certain molecules that facilitate this part of the process. These too must be present and active. If all the details are not correct, then problems can arise.

As an example, we will consider glucose. The hormone insulin has to be present in order to stimulate the cells' uptake of glucose. This means that your pancreas has to manufacture the insulin and secrete it on demand, a process that requires zinc. Once the insulin gets to the cells that need the glucose, another compound is necessary, called glucose tolerance factor or GTF. This contains chromium, the vitamin niacin and the sulphur-containing amino acid cysteine. Chromium, a trace mineral, is often in short supply in the diet and without it the cells may not be able to absorb the glucose they need, with the result that you will feel tired and your blood sugar levels will rise. The B vitamins, including niacin, are often lacking in a diet that contains lots of sugar and refined carbohydrates (precisely the diet for which you require large amounts of GTF to be present and to be exceptionally active). The cysteine may be in short supply if you don't eat eggs or sufficient quantities of certain other proteins.

In other words, this seemingly simple process of getting glucose into the cells so it can be used to produce energy, is dependent on a number of vitamins and minerals and, if these are not available, the process can go wrong and you will feel tired.

Cellular Energy Production

Virtually all reactions in the body need enzymes, biological catalysts that make the reactions possible, and coenzymes that help the enzymes. The enzymes are proteins made in the cells and the coenzymes are usually vitamins and minerals.

The next step is to convert the glucose and fatty acids that have entered the cells into energy. This process is done entirely within the cells and largely, though not entirely, within one type of organelle (or organ) within the cell, the mitochondria.

By now all the carbohydrate is in the form of glucose. This glucose goes through about twenty reactions within the cell. Each reaction requires that its enzyme and coenzymes are present. During the reaction sequence small quanta of energy are released until by the end of the process the glucose has been broken down into carbon dioxide and water plus little packets of energy which have been picked up and stored in small energy molecules called ATP.

Think back to the analogy we used earlier of rechargeable batteries. When a battery has lost its charge it corresponds to ADP. When it has been charged, (when it has had some energy added to it), it is equivalent to ATP. When, later on, it delivers its energy to wherever it is needed, it is reduced to ADP.[2] In the meantime this ATP is available, like a freshly charged battery, and can be called upon to deliver its small units of energy quickly wherever it is needed.

If all the batteries have been recharged, all the ADP has been converted into ATP, and there is still more glucose being broken down – in other words, if you have eaten too much for your immediate energy needs – something has to be done. The energy contained in the ATP has to be stored in some other way so that ADP is left and is available to pick up the energy still being released from your food. To achieve this, the spare ATP energy is used to build up fatty acids which are then stored (as anyone who has overeaten knows) in fat deposits, and you gain weight.

Fats are dealt with in much the same way as glucose. Individual fatty acids are broken down, through about twenty reactions, into carbon dioxide and water, and in the process energy is again released as fully-charged ATP molecules.

Amino acids are dealt with in a slightly different manner initially. The first use to which you put amino acids is to rebuild your own protein, your own muscles and organs. In addition, some amino acids are needed individually as specific messenger or communication molecules and as hormones. Any excess amino acids are 'spare', and are considered to be of no further use as amino acids. As a result, the 'amino' part is dealt with by the liver and released in the urine as ammonia, and the rest is 'burnt' for energy, just like the fatty acids and glucose,

Unfortunately, amino acids are not an efficient source of energy as about a third of the energy they produce is required to process them in the first place. It is also a strain on the liver and kidneys to have to process the excess ammonia you will generate if you rely on proteins for energy. So if you are looking for energy, focus on complex carbohydrates instead.

Notice that any spare energy is either delivered by ATP to wherever it is needed, or used to rebuild large fat molecules. These fats are the most compact and efficient way of storing energy. They end up on your hips, thighs, buttocks and stomach and, to a lesser extent, all over your body, and that is where you see them. Be glad they are fat molecules. If you were to store this energy as carbohydrates, they would take up even more space and make you look even bigger.

If you do not eat for a while and all the available fully-charged ATP molecules are used up, your body mobilises some of these stored fats and, as already indicated, delivers them to the cells that need energy. This in itself is a complex process depending on a variety of hormones and other messenger molecules. Once the fat reaches and enters the cells, it is burned up in the same way as if it came from food you had just eaten. In this way, you rebuild your level of ATP; you recharge the rundown ADP batteries into the fully-charged ATP batteries.

There is an important compound that is involved in this step of mobilising the fatty acids and making it possible for them to enter the cells. It is an amino acid called carnitine. This, as we shall see later (Chapter Five),

is made in your body from other amino acids derived
from protein foods. It is this carnitine that enables the
fat to enter the cells and to be available for combustion,
much as Glucose Tolerance Factor (GTF) enables glucose
to enter the cells. If you do not have sufficient carnitine,
there are serious consequences for your energy production that we will come back to later.

General

That's what should happen. Many substances are essential and have to come from the diet. Clearly, it is a
complex process. There's many a slip twixt cup and lip.
A lot can go wrong. The wonder is that problems do not
occur more often than they do.

In Part II you will find out some of the things that
can, and often do, go wrong with this process. You will
also discover how to correct them and to ensure that
you do, in future, get the system running properly and
release all the energy you need from your food.

[1] And with the help of appropriately-trained health care professionals.

[2] In case you are curious, ADP stands for Adenosine Di-Phosphate and
ATP for Adenosine Tri-Phosphate.

Chapter Two

Can Your Diet Supply Enough?

Many people, when trying to eat well, aim for the 'well-balanced diet' as if it is the answer to their problems. Others consider, wrongly, that they always do eat a balanced diet and so should not feel tired. What is the right balance, and does it supply all the nutrients you need?

I researched this and found the results dismaying. There are several different sets of instruction as to exactly how to create a well-balanced diet. I followed all of them, constructed a variety of diets according to the rules given and then analysed them for nutrient and calorie content. It soon became clear that none of them could provide all the nutrients needed, so I then used my knowledge of the (high) nutrient levels of specific individual foods and tried to create the best possible diet within these guidelines. It was still not possible to come up with one that contained the Recommended Daily Allowance (RDA)[1] of all the nutrients and remained within a calorie count to avoid weight gain. Since many nutritionists consider that even the RDA levels of nutrients are minimal levels and too low for optimum health, the problem is even worse than it might seem at first.

What Has to be Balanced?

You need approximately fifty to sixty nutrients, in the right proportions, for optimum health. This is what you need:

- **Amino acids**
  (a) iso-leucine, leucine, lysine, methionine, phenylalanine, threonine, tryptophan and valine.
  (b) arginine and histidine.
  (c) alanine, asparagine, cysteine, glutamic acid, glutamine, glycine, proline, serine, tyrosine.
  (d) carnitine, taurine.
- **Fatty acids**
  (a) linoleic acid and linolenic acid.
  (b) arachidonic acid.
- **Carbohydrate**
  (a) starch, the ideal source of glucose.
- **Vitamins**
  (a) Thiamine, riboflavin, niacin, pantothenic acid, pyridoxine, folic acid, cobalamine, PABA, biotin, ascorbic acid.
  (b) Vitamins A, D, E (and all the tocopherols) and K.
- **Minerals/elements**
  (a) sodium, potassium, calcium, magnesium, iron.
  (b) chromium, copper, manganese, molybdenum, selenium, silica, vanadium, zinc.
  (c) chlorine, fluoride, iodine, phosphorous, sulphur.
- **Nutritional factors**
  lecithin, choline, inositol.
  bioflavonoids, carotenes.
  carnitine.
- You also need fibre, water and air.

The Minimal Nutrient List

It is true that your body can make *some* of the above nutrient factors, *provided you are in optimum health and have enough of the correct ingredients for making them.* For instance,

If an adult has sufficient of the amino acids in group (a), they can make the others.

If a child has sufficient of the amino acids in groups (a) and (b), they can make all the others.

If you have sufficient linoleic acid, you can survive without the other two, although linolenic acid is highly protective for your heart and is an anti-inflammatory.

If you have adequate exposure to the sun, sufficient cholesterol and co-enzymes you can make your vitamin D in the skin.

If you have sufficient carotene and can break it down efficiently you can generate your own vitamin A.

If your liver is efficient and you have sufficient methionine, lysine, B group vitamins and linoleic acid you can make your own carnitine, choline and lecithin.

If your digestive system is totally healthy and you do not take antibiotics you (or the organisms within you) can make biotin, vitamin B12, some other B group vitamins and vitamin K within your own digestive system.

In this way, you can reduce the list of necessary nutrients somewhat. But do you want to give yourself the absolute minimum needs required by a body that is operating with maximum efficiency (and yours may not be); or do you want to be sure you have a plentiful supply of all nutrients and the best chance of maximum health and energy, taking into account your present state of health?

However you add them up, there are over forty nutrients you need, in adequate amounts on a daily basis. When you create and eat the well-balanced diet, you have to be sure that you are getting all of these, in adequate amounts. When you realise how many different nutrients you need, the ones that are absolutely essential for survival, plus the factors that can make the difference between good and poor health, the problem of getting all the nutrients you need, and in the right proportions, can seem overwhelming.

Because of the complexity and length of the list, it would be difficult to obtain your nutritional needs from processed foods. It is clearly much easier to get all these nutrients when you eat food just as it 'grows'. In other words, plants as they grow and animals as they move around in the wild, are biological systems, just as humans are. They either make for themselves (plants and animals), or take in from their environment in the form of food (animals) nutrients similar to the ones we, as humans, need. As a result, when we eat them, we acquire this wide range of compounds.

The plants take up raw materials from their environment, including minerals, and build an amazing variety of complex organic compounds. These compounds include the fats, proteins and carbohydrates you need for energy, and the vitamins required to access this energy. These plants are then eaten by the animals that can only make a few of these substances for themselves and who use the plants and make other nutrients from them such as the carnitine already mentioned. This means that if you eat fresh plant foods and recently-killed animal foods, you will get the maximum nutrient intake possible from foods grown by current agricultural practices.

As soon as you start processing food in any way, the nutrient level drops and the level of unwanted additives increases. Your choice of the less nutritious foods is affected by a number of factors.

- Your taste buds have almost certainly been so strongly influenced by the various flavours, flavour enhancers, texture modifiers, salt, sugar and other substances added to foods, that it would be unwise to rely on instinct to guide your choice of food and expect it to provide what your body needs.
- You have been heavily influenced by advertising and your own family tradition, by the social implications of certain foods and by your emotional attachments to particular types of food.
- You have to consider – how little time you have to buy and prepare food, how much time you can afford for eating.
- The financial considerations can throw a spanner in the works, as it often seems that the better-quality or more nutritious foods are too expensive. In fact it is much cheaper, overall, to eat unprocessed foods than processed foods. In addition the negative health and energy consequences of eating seemingly 'cheap' food are often enough to destroy your budget for life.

For all these reasons, the rules that define the well-balanced diet, inadequate as they are, have been formulated. No one, as I discovered, no matter how good their diet seems to be, actually follows them or sticks to them. Of the thousands of patients I have seen over the years, none has had an eating pattern that is as good as the defined diet and most people's eating pattern is a lot worse.

The Rules

There are several sets of rules for creating the well-balanced diet and they can be found in standard books on nutrition. The four food group system is based on:

1 Fresh meats, eggs, beans, lentils and nuts (plus other seeds such as sunflower, sesame) – two or more servings.
2 Dairy products – two to four cups of milk or equivalent, depending on age.
3 Grains – four or more servings.
4 Fruit and vegetables – at least six servings every day.

The five food group system is the same as that given above with the addition of a fifth group, namely:

5 Other: fats such as butter, oil and margarine.

Since it was recognised that neither of these plans provided adequate nutrition, the seven food group system was developed, namely:

1 Meat, fish, poultry – two servings of 3 oz
2 Legumes and/or nuts – two servings = 1 cup (legumes) or $1/2$ cup (nuts)
3 Milk – two servings milk or milk products
4 Fruits and vegetables – four servings
5 Whole grain products – four servings
6 Fat or oil – One serving (for vitamin E)
7 Others

While this provides increased levels of nutrients, it *still* does not reach RDA levels. It also introduces a problem. If you eat this amount on a daily basis you will gain weight rapidly, thus generating other health problems.

Furthermore, there is *no* room in these plans for *any* sugar, alcohol, fat-rich foods, etc, and the moment you add these in, as virtually everyone does, the average nutrient content of the diet falls even further.

The Two Food Group System – The Caveman Diet

When in doubt, it is worth casting an eye over history. For millions of years, our ancestors ate what they could hunt, scavenge or gather, as they wandered nomadically across the continents. This meant that their food consisted of:

1 Fresh meats and fish, eggs, nuts and protein-rich seeds.
2 Fruit and vegetables.

No wild animal will stand around waiting to be milked, so the 'dairy products' group was unavailable. Wild grasses yield very few seeds and make dry eating if you don't cook them. So until humans settled long enough in once place for the development of agriculture and traditional cooking habits, the 'grains' were not a significant part of the diet. Were our ancestors, by relying on food from only two groups, not getting all the nutrition they needed? Or were they, in fact, eating a diet that we would do well to emulate?

It is interesting to note here that, even if our ancient ancestors did eat the seeds of wild grasses, the 'grains' they were eating were very different from the ones we consume today. It is thought that during the processes that have changed them from wild to cultivated grasses, the protein content of the seed has fallen markedly, possibly from as high as 28% or more, to our present relatively low protein content, generally in the range of 6–12%, while the carbohydrate content has risen. This would mean that the breads of our recent ancestors, the 'staple food,' was very different from what it is today, not only in vitamin, mineral and fibre content but in protein content as well, and that where once it may have deserved its place in the centre of the diet, this is no longer true.

It is also interesting to note that these foods that have been introduced into our diet relatively recently – the grains and dairy products – are foods to which people with allergies commonly react. People are much less likely to be allergic to the foods that fall within the two food groups that comprised the diet of our earlier ancestors. We will discuss this further later (Chapter Eighteen).

I created a variety of diets along the two food group basis. The results were mildly encouraging. The overall nutrient content was significantly higher than that of the other diets but it was still unable to provide the full RDA level of all the nutrients within an appropriate calorie intake. The assumption inherent in the definition of the RDA is that if you start out one-hundred-per-cent fit and healthy, not only without any symptoms but with exuberant good health, and you consume the RDA of each nutrient specified, every single day, then you should remain healthy.

Summary

From this it is clear that a well-balanced-diet does *not* provide all the nutrients you need, even if you are totally healthy and absolutely symptom-free, as assumed in the RDA concept. If you have any symptoms, however mild, the situation will be even worse since your nutrient needs increase as your health deteriorates. If you are tired now, then certainly the RDA levels, by definition, are not sufficient and the well balanced diet is even more inadequate for you.

How Does This Come About?

On the face of it, this seems an extraordinary conclusion to reach – that you cannot get all the nutrients you need for exuberant good health and energy from the best possible diet you can create from twentieth-century food. The conclusion is accurate; the problem lies in the last three words, 'twentieth-century food'.

If we look carefully at the changes that have taken place during recent centuries, and particularly during recent decades, we find that the quality of our diets – their nutrient content – has decreased, often quite dramatically At the same time we have been exposed to an increasing number of toxins, chemicals, radiation, other physical hazards and other challenges to our health, all of which mean we actually need additional nutrients for protection. In other words, our nutrient requirements have increased and the quantity we are actually getting (if we don't take supplements) has decreased.

The nutrient level of your food has gone *down* for a variety of reasons:

1 Farmed food generally contains less nutrients than food grown wild – as herbalists know.
2 Food grown on the same ground year after year gradually depletes the soil of nutrients – nutrients essential for us, if not for the plant's survival.
3 Modern fertilisers render a lot of the trace minerals in the soil unavailable to the plants.
4 Vine-ripened fruits and vegetables have more nutrients than those picked early. Early picking may

be necessary for easy transport and storage, but it does reduce the level of nutrients you receive.

5 When you eat the flesh from animals that have run wild, you get a large proportion of protein and a small amount of fat, a high proportion of it unsaturated. When you eat the flesh of domesticated animals that have had little to do all day except eat and sleep, you get less protein and a lot more fat. Further, the fat that you do get is a lot more saturated than the fat from wild animals.

6 Vitamins are delicate substances, easily damaged by heat, light, by acids or alkalis and by storage. Inevitably they start to breakdown as soon as you either store or process the food.

All this means that even if you eat only fresh, unprocessed foods, your diet is likely to be less nutritious, less rich in vitamins and minerals, than the best diets available a few centuries or even decades ago.

Very few people eat only fresh, unprocessed foods. Most people eat a lot of processed foods – from breads (processed grains) to smoked and cured meats, from jams to soft drinks, from chocolates to ice-cream and from tins and bottles of sauces and flavourings to tinned or frozen 'instant' meals. A few people consciously aim to eat a good and unprocessed diet, but even when they are trying their best, other foods sneak in from time to time. They may come when you eat out, or when you allow yourself small additions to your unprocessed diet for a treat or for convenience. Each time these additions occur, the overall nutrient-content of your diet diminishes. You may argue that you only slip up occasionally, that no one can be perfect all the time. This may be so, but given the gradual erosion of the quality of your diet, by myriad small steps until, without quite realising it, you are indeed eating a diet considerably deficient in nutrients, you will certainly benefit from taking nutritional supplements.

Your nutrient requirement has *risen* for a variety of reasons. Nearly every facet of modern living, from the mere fact of living in an urban environment to the increasing demands for the perceived benefits of high technology, exerts a challenge on your body and your health. To counter this challenge you need *more* nutrients than your ancestors, not less. Here are some examples, just a very few of the thousands that could be given.

- Chlorine in the drinking water increases your need for all antioxidants, especially vitamin E.
- Lead in petrol fumes increases the need for zinc and calcium.
- Pollution in general and cigarette smoke in particular increases your need for vitamin A, zinc, vitamin C and lecithin.
- Antibiotics reduce your ability to make the B group of vitamins and vitamin K via the organisms in your small intestines.
- The contraceptive pill increases the need for vitamin B6 in particular and a number of vitamins plus zinc, magnesium and manganese in general.
- Stress increases enormously your body's need for all nutrients.

Other factors that damage the body and increase its need for nutrients for repair and prevention include:

- The thousands of chemicals in food from farm chemicals such as growth enhancers, pesticides, and herbicides to the colours, flavours, stabilisers and preservatives that are added as part of the processing.

- Medical drugs all have side effects, and all increase the need for protective nutrients. Many of them have specific actions on certain nutrients.
- Social drugs – alcohol, coffee and tea – are diuretic and increase nutrient loss in the urine.
- Cigarettes and recreational drugs increase the body's nutritional needs in many ways.
- Physical factors greatly increase the need for nutrients to protect the body from the harm they cause. These include radiation; increased exposure to ozone (both at ground level and even more so when flying); computer screens; the entire electromagnetic spectrum including radio and television waves that permeates our environment, unseen, all the time; fluorescent lights and air conditioning.
- Televisions are also a problem. A colleague described the case of a young boy who became hyperactive when his bed was moved against the wall backing on to the television in the sitting-room; his parents moved the television and he recovered.

The Result

The changes in farming and food-processing practices over the centuries explains how it has come about that today's diet, even the so-called well-balanced diet, will not provide you with a fully adequate amount of all the nutrients you need. The potentially lethal combination of reduced nutrient intake *and* increased nutrient needs puts your health, your energy and your well-being at risk. It is no wonder that the incidence of nutritionally-related health problems, including fatigue, both general and chronic, has risen rapidly over the past few decades and now accounts for well over fifty per cent of all deaths. We have now reached the stage where even some medical practitioners attest to this fact.

What To Do

Be thankful that the modern technology that has reduced the nutrient level of much of our farm produce and further reduced the levels of nutrients in processed foods, and that has created so much that is damaging to our health, has also provided the technology that has enabled us to understand the individual nutrients and their role in the body and the ability to extract or manufacture these nutrients and provide them in concentrated form, as supplements.

If you are tired, it could well be because you are not getting sufficient nutrients – either because of decreased supply or because of increased need, or both. This concept will come up again and again throughout the book in relation to your need for more energy. If you are reluctant to take supplements I hope you will reassess your views in the light of this chapter.

If you do feel that supplements are important, I hope this chapter has helped to reinforce your view. You may also need some of the above information when other people try to persuade you that taking supplements is a waste of time, or an exercise in creating expensive urine. (This is nonsense since before the nutrients are expelled in urine, they have been deployed all round your body, doing their job in a variety of cells. You wouldn't tell a housewife there was no need for her to shop for food simply because she puts a rubbish bin of used and spent material out each week.) Some people continue to argue that because people did not take, or possibly did not need to take, supplements in the past, they should not do so now. Yet this is inconsistent with attitudes to other aspects of life. You do not refuse to use a motor car or public transport because they are not the way your grandparents and great grandparents got about. You do not refuse to use electric lights because for millennia flames were used. You do not refuse to wear clothes made of modern fabrics because they are not the same as the furs and skins your ancestors wore. In the same way, I suggest you rethink any possible unwillingness to take nutritional supplements because it is not the old way of doing things.

Just as you are happy or compelled to be exposed to the harm and damage to your body caused by our present level of high technology, so too it is appropriate to appreciate and utilise what this same level of high technology and understanding has enabled us to do in providing nutritional supplements that help counter the damage this technology has caused us and so to protect our health.

Conclusion

In this chapter it has become clear that, in the twentieth or twenty-first century, living within the effects of technology and consuming the foods of commerce, you are unlikely to get all the nutrients you need for one-hundred-per-cent, exuberant health and abundant energy from your diet, and a blind, head-in-the-sand assumption that you will could well be behind your tiredness and lack of energy.

As you read the rest of this book, keep this in mind. Keep it in mind when we consider the role each of the nutrients plays in generating the energy you want. Keep it in mind when we consider the various health problems that may sap your energy or increase your need for energy and the way individual nutrients can help with these problems. Above all, keep it in mind when we consider Chronic Fatigue Syndrome (CFS) and the way nutrient deficiencies can reduce the function of your immune system. This in turn affects the way your body copes with the toxins and stressors that have led to the overload and breakdown that is part of this syndrome.

The Energy Equation

Since you are primarily concerned with the amount of energy you have, or have not, got, there is a final fact to consider in this chapter: the energy equation. The energy equation is simple. In normal health, where you are neither gaining nor losing weight and where you have sufficient energy to do all you want, it is:

ENERGY IN (from   =   ENERGY OUT (available for
food and nutrients)   repair and activity)

However, for you to have all the energy that is potentially available from the macronutrients you eat, the fats, proteins and carbohydrates, the process must operate efficiently. In other words:

ENERGY IN = ENERGY OUT
provided all the necessary micronutrients are available

If you are tired and, no matter what you eat, do not have sufficient energy, several things could be happening.

Under-supply
- You are eating insufficient quantity of food.
- You are eating sufficient quantity but not the right quality of foods; certain nutrients are missing.
- You are eating the right foods but not absorbing all the nutrients, for a variety of reasons.
- There is some block in the conversion of this fuel (food) to energy.
- Or any combination of these.

Increased requirements
- You are trying to do too much
- You have a health problem that is interfering with energy production.
- You have a health problem that is burning up energy faster than you are generating it.
- Or any combination of these.

We shall be considering these various possibilities in the next sections.

The production of energy can be crystallised by another equation:

$$\left.\begin{array}{c}\text{CARBOHYDRATES}\\ \text{and}\\ \text{FATS}\\ \text{and}\\ \text{PROTEINS}\end{array}\right\} + \text{OXYGEN} \rightarrow \left\{\begin{array}{l}\text{CARBON DIOXIDE which}\\ \text{goes to the LUNGS and}\\ \text{WATER which is expelled via}\\ \text{the kidneys as URINE and}\\ \text{ENERGY – which is our goal}\end{array}\right.$$

Again, all the micronutrients, the vitamins and minerals, *must* also be present for the appropriate amount of energy to be developed.[2]

[1] The RDA, or Recommended Daily Amount, has been formulated by the Food and Nutrition Board of the National Academy of Sciences in America. This body comprises a group of people involved in nutrition and health research and the food industry. The RDA is, in the opinion of the board, the amount of each nutrient required by most healthy people. Health, in this context, is defined, not only as the absence of symptoms but as a state of full mental and physical well-being. The RDA level of each nutrient is often inadequate for people who are not in perfect health. In addition, it is adequate for some but not for all healthy people. Thus even if you did get the RDA level of each nutrient you might still be undernourished measured against the yardstick of your own specific needs. If you are tired, or have Chronic Fatigue Syndrome, you will almost certainly need more.

[2] Detailed discussion of the topics discussed in this chapter and details of the diets, their analysis and nutrient levels are given in 'The Well-

Balanced-Diet' by Xandria Williams, in *Australian Wellbeing* No. 12, 1986; *What's In My Food* by Xandria Williams, Nature and Health Books, 1988. Both can be obtained from the author.

PART II

Generating Insufficient Energy

Fatigue is among the top ten reasons for seeing a health care professional, even though it may not be the first problem the patient discusses. For doctors, such complaints are frustrating as they have no drug or recognised medication to give to the patient to solve the problem of fatigue. This is hardly surprising as the problem is one of diet and lifestyle and its solution involves changes to diet and to lifestyle, plus nutritional changes and supplements; not the administration of a drug. The doctors' attitude often is that if you are not ill with something they can identify, then you must be well.

Yet in between total health and overt illness is this grey area of being just 'not well', of being tired, run down, lethargic, below par, not coping and so forth. This area often extends to include health problems such as hypoglycaemia, thrush, allergies and problems related to nutritional deficiencies or an excess of toxins. These problems leave you exhausted yet without an identifiable disease. For naturopaths and other natural or alternative therapists, problems without organic lesions do exist and can be dealt with readily. Their approach is not to look for a drug to 'fix' the problem, or to eliminate the overt symptoms, but rather to assume that a health problem comes from an inadequacy within your own body, an inadequacy that is generally the result of not providing the body with all that it needs. If these deficiencies can be identified and the body given all that it needs to put itself right, it can repair itself and restore normal working function. This is something your body is supremely good at doing, *provided* it is spared too many toxins *and* is given all the resources it needs in the way of nutrients and so forth.

Fatigue is also a recognised part of many specific organic diseases, so much so that most people expect to feel tired when they are unwell. Their body is spending all its available energy combating the disease process and there is little left for normal energetic activities. The disease process itself, as well as resulting in reduced energy, may actually have been caused by reduced energy and resources.

American studies have shown that about a quarter of patients going to their practitioner and complaining of fatigue have a chronic health problem such as malignancies, heart disease, anaemia and inflammatory problems. Over a third have mild diseases and over a third have no specific disease. Of those with no obvious specific diseases, about forty per cent are eventually found to have some associated physical problem; another forty per cent are tired as a result of psychological problems. About ten per cent have a combination of problems and in the remainder the cause is undetermined.

In this section, we will be considering the lack of energy that results when, through nutritional deficiencies at the cellular level, insufficient energy is generated for the normal daily needs of the individual. In Part III we shall consider energy problems in association with other physical health problems.

Chapter Three

How to Make Sure You Generate Normal Energy

In the previous Section (Chapter One), I outlined the normal stages in energy production from choosing the food to digesting it, absorbing it, transporting it into the cells and converting it into energy. I assumed everything was happening the way it should. This is rarely the case, so it is time now to find out what commonly goes wrong and how to correct the situations that arise as a result.

Just to remind you, here are the steps, plus a few new ones, all of which should occur correctly.   How do you rate?

- Correct choice of food, for maximum nutritional content.
- Nutrient-saving preparation of the food.
- Correct and full breakdown of this food in the digestive tract.
- Efficient absorption of these components across the intestinal wall and into the bloodstream.
- Proper transport of these nutrients through the bloodstream to every cell in the body.
- Easy uptake of these nutrients by the individual cells.
- Correct biochemical breakdown of the

macronutrients via the metabolic pathways within the cell.

- Efficient short term storage of the energy released, in high energy molecules.
- Ready availability of these high energy compounds as needed.
- Correct storage of excess energy in long-term energy storage molecules.
- Availability of this stored energy as needed.

Before you read Chapter One and the above sequence, it seemed easy, didn't it? It seemed that all you had to do was to eat the food you chose (on the basis of budget, taste, convenience or custom) or were given, and that as a result you generated the energy you needed and could get on with your life with no further concerns. Now it is clear that the process is much more complicated than that. The good news is that when you are well all these complications and details are dealt with at the subconscious level by your wise body. The bad news is that when you don't give the body the raw materials it needs and don't look after it properly, this body lets you know that it is now the turn of your conscious mind. This conscious mind, triggered by the pain, tiredness and discomfort that arise from faulty metabolism, is going to have to learn more about health and nutrition and to make some decisions about the changes that must be made to restore (a) your body to health and (b) the process to one that can occur unconsciously again with no further disturbance in the way of symptoms.

For many people, recognising all the steps that have to be accomplished (and that can go wrong) makes a lack of energy seem less simple and more worthy of attention to all the details than when they were less well informed. This is the part that seems to make all the difference to patients. Once they understand the details, they are more willing to do whatever it takes to put the process right than when they are simply given the instructions like a set of rules.

Don't worry, you are not going to be taken through a full biochemical description of what happens. The following general guide will be sufficient.

1. Correct Choice of Food, for Maximum Nutritional Content

It is up to you to make the correct decisions about the food you will eat. To make these decisions, you require some knowledge. Below is a simple guide to help you on your way.

Do eat or consume	*Instead of*
Fresh fruits and vegetables, preferably organically grown	Frozen, dried or tinned fruits and vegetables
100% wholemeal bread	White bread; grain bread, that is cracked grains in a white flour bread base; commercial 'wholemeal breads' made with sifted wholemeal flour or added white flour
Rolled oats or raw mueslies	Processed breakfast cereals
Wholemeal pasta	White pasta, green or coloured pasta
Brown rice	White or yellow rice
Fresh fish	Fish that is frozen, tinned or smoked; fish fingers; fish pâtés or processed fish products
Lean chicken	Pressed chicken; chicken sausages; chicken skin
Lean meat as cut from the carcass	Sausages, processed meats, smoked meats
Fresh liver	Liver pâté

Raw or pasteurised milk	Homogenised milk
Cottage cheese	Cream cheese
Natural cheeses	Cheese slices and cheese spreads
Butter	Margarine
Plain yoghurt	Flavoured yoghurt and yoghurt-style deserts
Fresh eggs, preferably free-range	Dried eggs or processed egg products
Raw nuts	Roasted nuts, whether salted or not
Dried beans, home-cooked	Tinned beans in sauces
Purified water	City drinking water
Mineral water	Soft drinks
Pure fruit juices	Fruit juice drinks, with added sugar
Fresh or dried herbs	Commercial flavourings
Spices	Commercial flavour enhancers
Cold-pressed oils	Commercially extracted oils
Oil and vinegar dressings	Commercial mayonnaise and salad dressings
Herb teas	Tea
Dandelion coffee or cereal beverages	Coffee, whether decaffeinated or not
Good quality wine in moderation (if you must!)	Cheap wines, beer, spirits and mixers, cola, tonic, ginger ale etc.
	Sweet liqueurs, cocktails

Do

Where possible, choose organically-grown grains, fruit and vegetables, free-range eggs, and milk and meat from animals reared on organic farms.

Buy fresh food and avoid food that has been kept in storage.

Avoid

Sugar and processed food products containing sugar. Honey is only slightly better than sugar and should only be eaten in moderation if at all.

Chocolates, lollies and candy bars.

Sweets, puddings and desserts other than those made from fresh fruit, plain yoghurt and whole grains.

White flour and anything made with it, including things listed above, plus pizzas, thickened soups, sauces, cakes, biscuits, buns, cookies, desserts.

Saturated animal fats such as cream, lard and the fat or skin on meats; fried foods and foods in batter. Butter is preferable to margarine but should only be used in moderation.

Salt and heavily-salted foods and condiments such as yeast-based spreads, sauces, salted pickles: read the labels.

Pre-cooked or pre-prepared meals complete with sauces and batters, whether frozen, tinned or dried.

Soup and gravy mixes.

Tinned foods.

Take-away hot foods that have been cooked and then kept hot.

Take-away foods high in fats and refined carbo-hydrates – and unfortunately this includes nearly all of them.

This may seem like a long list of 'don'ts' and a short list of 'do's. It is. This in itself is a clear reflection, if one is needed, of the amount of poor-quality food that is available, promoted and sold. No wonder so many people are undernourished and overtired.

2. Nutrient-saving Preparation of the Food

The next step is to prepare the food in such a way that you save the maximum amount of the nutrients it contains. Obviously the ideal scenario – the one that leads to the maximum delivery of nutrients – is for you to pick fruits and vegetables when they are ripe and eat them raw and on the spot. This way, they will deliver their maximum nutrient potential. Post-picking deterioration will be at a minimum. However, in these days of urban living this is rarely possible, practical or convenient.

We will assume you have chosen foods from the left-hand column above. Buy food as fresh as possible, from a fruit and vegetable market rather than pre-packaged foods that may have been sitting in the supermarket cooler. Buy fresh produce in small quantities, take it home and eat it within a day or two. Storing food for days, whether in the refrigerator or not, allows the nutrient content to decrease further.

Eat food *raw* as much as possible. There is rarely a need to cook fruit. When ripe, it is already soft and ready to eat. Cooking it only turns it into a mush and depletes its nutrient content. There are many interesting and exciting dishes you can make with fruits without having to cook them. If you want their flavour in a hot savoury dish then add them at the very last minute and give them just sufficient time to warm up.

Vegetables should be eaten raw as salads as often as possible, rather than cooked. Salads do not consist solely of lettuce, cucumber and tomato. You can eat almost any vegetable raw in a salad. A friend introduced me to a salad of raw grated parsnip with fresh lemon juice squeezed over it: delicious. Fresh and grated beetroot is preferable to tinned, pickled and sweetened beetroot. Raw corn, cut off the cob, is tasty and nutritious. Grated pumpkin, chopped cauliflower and broccoli, sliced onions – these and many other vegetables can make a delightful salad, either as a main meal or as a side dish.

If you are making a salad to take to work for lunch, cut the vegetables into large pieces rather than grating them. The greater the exposed surface area, the greater the nutrient loss due to oxidation. For the same reason, foods should be chopped and prepared immediately before you need them for eating or cooking, not chopped and then left to stand.

When cooking, cook only as much as you will eat. One patient told me proudly that he had eaten fresh vegetables all week. In view of his previous disinclination either to eat salads or cook, and his preferred diet of steak and chips, I was impressed, until he let me know that he cooked up a huge pot of vegetables every Sunday and then reheated it each evening until it was finished on the Saturday night. By the end of the week, its nutrient content would have been minimal.

Vegetables should be only lightly cooked, not overcooked: they should still have some crunch in them. They will keep their maximum nutrient content if they are steamed. Do not use aluminium ware: then, if you cook them in a centimetre or so of water, you can use this water as a gravy. Another flavoursome method is to line a casserole dish with thinly-sliced onion (this sweats and means you do not have to use fat or water to prevent the other vegetables sticking), then lay all the other vegetables, on top cut to suitable sizes so that they will all cook in the same length of time, put on the lid and place in a moderate oven. Allow them to cook until they are just soft enough to eat.

Meat is best if cooked for a long time at a low temperature. This can be done in a crock pot. Another excellent way to do this is to put the meat in the oven at around 275°F or 135°C for sufficient time to kill surface bacteria, then reduce the temperature to around 150°F or 70°C and give it three times the normal cooking time to complete. Even once it is cooked, no harm will come to it if it is left in the oven for a longer period – so you can put this in the oven in the morning, knowing that when you come home at night it will be ready to eat. It will be a lot more juicy, tender and tasty than meat that has been cooked more rapidly. Furthermore, there is less vitamin loss since the greatest loss occurs at high temperatures; much less occurs at low temperatures, even allowing for the extra cooking time. Finish by raising the temperature again just prior to serving.

If you must cook meats quickly, do so in such a way as to keep them as moist as possible and above all, avoid fat, particularly burnt, blackened or crackling fat. The heat required to burn the fats increases the chances of carcinogenic compounds being formed within the fat.

Once food is cooked, eat it as soon as it has cooled to a comfortable temperature. It is unwise to eat food that is almost too hot to touch.

Ideally, whole grains and seeds should be ground as and when you need them. You can do small amounts in a coffee grinder. But if this is not practical buy a small amount of flour at a time and don't plan to keep it for too long.

Certainly, it takes more time to cook 'from scratch' than to buy pre-prepared foods, cooked beans in tins, pre-made sauces, tinned soups and so forth, and heat them in the microwave, but the health and energy benefits of cooking from scratch are significant. The extra energy you gain from good eating will actually give you more spare time to do things, even allowing for the extra amount of time spent on food preparation.

3. Correct Breakdown of Food in the Digestive Tract

Digestion starts in the mouth. It is very important that you *chew* your food thoroughly. Ideally, this should be fifty times a mouthful but few people manage anything near that. However, try it once, as an experiment. You will find that grains, for instance, become progressively sweeter as the starches are broken down into sugar, the maltose mentioned earlier (Chapter One). Some foods, such as fruits, make this impossible, but experiment with more chewing time. Since the only place you have taste buds is in your mouth, you might as well keep the food there as long as you can and enjoy the flavours. After all, you were probably looking forward to eating it as much for the taste as for its satiety value.

If you don't chew, out of laziness, then you can change this by a conscious decision. On the other hand, you may have problems in the mouth that make chewing difficult or painful: sore gums, problems such as mouth ulcers, a painful tongue or ill-fitting dentures. These problems should be remedied as they can lead to poor digestion, poor nutrition and fatigue due to low nutrient levels, and also to a variety of other health problems. In addition, the mere fact that you have these problems in your mouth is a sign that there are deeper problems you should be correcting.

If your tongue is ridged, sore, beefy or inflamed, you may be short of a number of the B group vitamins. If your taste buds have lost their sensitivity (or if you find yourself complaining frequently that foods don't taste as good as they used to), you could be short of zinc or vitamin C. A lack of vitamin C and the bioflavonoids can lead to spongy and painful gums and, eventually, the teeth becoming loose and even falling out. The teeth themselves need not only calcium but a variety of minerals including magnesium, zinc, manganese, copper, silica plus other trace nutrients such as fluoride (in small amounts). If you do not get all these nutrients, you are likely to have tooth cavities, and teeth that break or become rotten as you get older. Without vitamin C and a variety of other nutrients that boost the immune system, you may also get infections in the teeth and gums. If you have any of these signs then it would be wise to take the appropriate action and correct your diet.

If you have already lost your teeth, or some of them, and have to wear a plate, then make sure it fits well. Of the people who need dentures, up to ten per cent decide to do without them; around thirty per cent should have them checked or corrected as they fit badly. People who wear dentures, particularly but not exclusively poorly-fitted dentures, do not chew their food properly. Worse, they often choose soft, overcooked food or highly-processed foods to make things easier in the mouth. These foods are usually much less nutritious than those that require chewing.

Even if you do choose and eat good foods, fresh fruits and vegetables and so forth, you will still have problems if you don't or can't chew properly. You cannot get all the nutrients out of food that goes down the tubes in large chunks and defies complete chemical breakdown later on, simply because of its size.

Relax when you eat. If you are angry, upset, frightened or worried, eat later. You know how dry your mouth gets when you are worried or angry. This means that not only is there less saliva production but there is also less production of digestive enzymes when you are tense than when you are relaxed. This in turn means that there is little point in forcing food down since it won't be properly digested and assimilated anyway. If you do have to eat when tense, then do all you can to relax, at least temporarily. Put other thoughts from your mind while you are eating. Make a conscious effort to relax your shoulders, relax your chest and, most importantly, relax the muscles of your abdomen.

Don't drink fluids when you eat, as these dilute the digestive juices. If you feel you simply have to drink to get the food down, then this should alert you to the fact that your digestive system may need some help: read on, as we shall be discussing this later. However, there is some evidence that a glass of wine with meals increases the flow of digestive juices; but only one glass – drink more and you start diluting these same digestive juices.

As people get older, and certainly by the time they are near or in their forties, it is not uncommon to find that the stomach cells have slowed down and that the production of hydrochloric acid has diminished. It is important that you do all you can to prevent this happening. The production of hydrochloric acid requires a number of the B group vitamins which you can take as part of your supplement programme. There are also tissues salts, available from most health foods shops, that can help, particularly Nat Mur and Kali Mur. Otherwise you can take a hydrochloric acid supplement in tablet form. This should be taken at the end of meals. Allow your own stomach acid to work on the first part of the meal and take the supplement to finish the job off.

If you burp, get a full feeling under your rib cage when you have eaten, or feel that you are not digesting food properly and it is just 'sitting there', you may be short of stomach acids. However it is equally possible that you won't have any obvious symptoms of the problem. There are several tests you can do to check this, but a simple one involves taking a supplement of hydrochloric acid and stomach enzymes with the end of your meal and noting if there is an improvement in your general symptoms and sense of well-being.

Do not be worried about having too much acid. Even

if you have an ulcer, it is not the amount of acid that is at fault. The acid is *meant* to be there and it is *supposed* to be so strong that if you were to put your finger (or a piece of the muscle wall of your stomach) in it it would disintegrate – just as a piece of steak would. To protect the muscle wall of your stomach from this acid, you have a mucilaginous layer that is impervious to the acid. If you feel pain, it is probable that this mucilaginous layer is damaged and needs to be repaired, but that is another story. Note that your stomach is situated tucked under your left rib cage, not in your abdomen where so many people commonly place it.

Other digestive problems can occur in the small intestine. The small intestine sits within your abdomen, where many people believe their 'stomach' to be. If you feel bloated here, it may because of some of the problems that we have already mentioned; problems that started higher up in your digestive system but which inevitably have consequences further down the tubes. It may also be because you have the wrong type of organisms in the intestines. One example of this is *candida albicans*, the organism involved in thrush. We will be considering that one later (Chapter Sixteen). Suffice it to say, if you have any digestive problems you should have them diagnosed and fixed. They may be part of the reason why you feel tired.

The final section of the digestive tract is the colon, the part where the waste material is processed ready for elimination. Again, if there are problems here, they should be fixed. Slippery elm powder and aloe vera juice are excellent at respectively soothing and protecting the walls of the digestive tract and encouraging them to heal. In fact, these two substances can help the whole digestive tract if there is damage, ulceration or pain.

Irritable bowel, spastic colon, diverticulitis and other colon problems can all lead to the production of toxins in the bowel. These toxins can then be absorbed into the bloodstream, flow through the body, and contribute to fatigue and lassitude. These are problems that can be dealt with relatively simply.

If you are constipated (less than three soft, bulky motions a day), the problems are likely to be worsened. There will be more toxins and more sluggishness. If you suffer from diarrhoea (liquid and very frequent bowel motions), then it is possible that nutrients are passing through too rapidly and are not being absorbed. This too can lead to fatigue. The ideal is to have three or four soft and bulky bowel motions a day, or about one after each time you eat. They should pass easily and quickly, be formed (just) and probably best described as 'mushy', not the hard lumps that most people seem to consider normal.

A word of warning is in order here. Over the years I have had hundreds of patients tell me after a week or two of the changes that we have instigated in their life-style, that they have diarrhoea, when in fact, they are having normal motions, possible for the first time in their adult lives.

4. Efficient Absorption of these Nutrients from the Intestine into the Bloodstream

One last step of digestion occurs on the intestinal walls, namely the breakdown of the disaccharides into their component monosaccharides. Apart from that, most of the activity at this point involves the transport of nutrients across the intestinal wall and into the bloodstream.

To achieve this, a number of mechanisms have to happen correctly. For some of the nutrients, particularly the minerals, there are specific carrier molecules that are necessary to transport them from the intestine into the bloodstream. These mechanisms are further complicated

by the fact that there are a variety of nutrients that
compete with each other for some of these carriers. Problems in this area are hard to detect, even by specialists
in this field of nutritional medicine, but you should
know that they can and do exist and could be contributing to your fatigue.

So many patients say, 'But I eat the right foods, I take
supplements. Why am I not healthy?' It is important that
you understand that there are many steps along the
way and that just because you have taken, say, a simple
multivitamin and a multimineral and improved your
diet, you have not necessarily done all you can on the
nutritional front.

It is extremely important to consider the details and
the overall health of the intestinal tract. In the chapter
on candidiasis (Chapter Sixteen), you will discover the
havoc that can be wrought on your health by the presence and activity of some moulds in your digestive tract.
There is also the harm that can be done by having other
pathogens there.

From the outside, the problem of 'wind' may seem
trivial, if somewhat embarrassing. On the inside, it
means that sections of your intestines are being 'blown
up' or bloated, and the walls are being stretched. This,
combined with the activity of the organisms causing the
problem and the toxins generated by these organisms,
can damage the intestine walls to the extent proper
assimilation of food is reduced.

Inflammatory problems in the intestines can reduce
nutrient absorption and increase fatigue. Weight loss
may occur through decreased absorption of nutrients
combined with possible loss of blood. Chron's disease
and ulcerative colitis are debilitating diseases and may
need expert attention. However, you can also do things
yourself.

There are many things you can do to improve the

situation and it is time to reiterate the main points. I make no apology for the fact that are many instructions repeated over and over again in this book. It will underline the fact that proper nutritional steps have multiple beneficial impacts throughout the body, your health in general and the production of energy in particular, and that when you 'cheat', when you fail to eat the foods that are good for you and fail to digest and absorb them properly, many health problems can and will result, including fatigue.

What You Can Do

- A high-fibre diet is important, as is proper chewing of food, the availability of adequate stomach acids, resting while you eat, and consuming a high nutrient diet, probably with the addition of supplements (see Chapter Two).
- Relax when you eat, chew the food thoroughly and do not drink while you eat.
- A teaspoon of slippery elm powder, either stirred into a liquid or mashed into a banana or some other food, two or three times a day, can put an 'internal bandage' on any painful or ulcerated area in the digestive tract, and
- Aloe vera juice, vitamins A and E and zinc can all assist the healing process, combined with overall good nutrition.
- Glutamine, an amino acid, has also been found to have a healing effect on the digestive tract.
- Take some correctly prepared and stored acidophilus and bifidus organisms to help the 'good guys' get re-established and crowd out the unwanted organisms.
- If it is appropriate, take a supplement containing stomach acid and digestive enzymes and another containing intestinal digestive enzymes.

5. Transport of these Nutrients through the Bloodstream to Every Cell in the Body

All being well, you have now fully digested the food you have eaten and it is ready for absorption. So let's see what happens next.

The macronutrients are transported relatively easily through the blood stream. Glucose (from the starches and simple sugars) and amino acids (from protein) are water-soluble and the fatty acids travel, combined with protein and cholesterol, in specially-prepared packages called lipoproteins. These lipoproteins vary in nature from high density to low density and it is the relative proportions of these that are important in preventing heart attacks. You want more of the high density variety and less of the low density variety. We will be talking about the heart, these lipoproteins and your energy levels later (Chapter Nineteen).

The water-soluble vitamins can also travel relatively easily through the bloodstream, as they dissolve readily. The fat-soluble vitamins have greater difficulty since the blood is aqueous. They commonly travel with the help of carrier molecules and yet other nutrients may be necessary for the formation of these carrier molecules. For instance, vitamin A is carried by retinol-binding protein, and zinc is necessary for its production, release and activity. As a result, a lack of zinc could cause an apparent vitamin A deficiency problem but it would not be resolved by taking a vitamin A supplement, only by taking a zinc supplement. Iron and copper are carried by iron-binding and copper-binding proteins respectively and their chemistry is closely interrelated (see Chapter Nine).

6. Proper Uptake of these Nutrients by the Cells

You may feel that we have already come a long way, but it is not yet time to relax. It is not sufficient to digest the food, absorb the nutrients and transport them, via the bloodstream, to the target cells. They still have to enter the cells, and even here there are important steps that must happen correctly.

Carnitine

The fatty acids, for instance, can be in the bloodstream but a specific set of reactions has to happen before they can enter the cells and be broken down and used as raw material in the production (or release) of energy. An amino acid called carnitine is necessary for the transport of the fatty acids into the cells. Two other amino acids, lysine and methionine, are necessary for the manufacture of carnitine. Other trace nutrients are needed as coenzymes for this process, particularly vitamin B6.

Now here comes the interesting part. Just like the vitamins, both lysine and methionine have to be obtained from your diet; you cannot make them in your body. The major dietary sources of methionine and lysine are meat and other animal products. Animal products are usually high in fats but hopefully you have sufficient carnitine to transfer fats into the cells. If, on the other hand, you are a vegetarian, and eat a diet with a relatively high fat content, including such things as nuts, mayonnaise, avocados, oils and so forth, it is possible to have 'hungry cells' bathed in a bloodstream that is rich with fatty acids but, because your diet is relatively low in lysine and methionine, lacking the carnitine necessary to get the fats into the cells. Thus you may feel tired and resort to eating which will, in all probability, continue to prolong the cycle and fail to generate the required energy.

The irony continues. If you are overweight and you go on a diet, you are effectively going on a high-fat regime. Half your food comes in via your mouth; the other half of the food energy is being supplied (you hope) by the mobilisation and utilisation of your stored body fat. Again, if you are a vegetarian and short of methionine and lysine, and hence of carnitine, this fat may try to enter the cells, fail to find the necessary carrier molecule and then return to the fat stores in disgust. You will then be a tired and frustrated, overweight vegetarian who yet again has failed to stick to a diet or lose weight successfully.

Chromium

Another problem with the cellular uptake of the macronutrients involves chromium and the uptake of sugar. When you eat a meal with a high sugar content, or one that includes refined white flour or white rice which breaks down rapidly to glucose, then your blood sugar level rises significantly. To bring that back down to normal, the hormone insulin is released from the pancreas and this encourages the cells to take up the glucose. The cells will then either use this glucose for energy production or, if none is needed, they will convert it into fats and send them off to the storage depots.

In this process, insulin does not act on its own. It needs a molecule called Glucose Tolerance Factor or GTF. This helps the insulin to do its job, and without it your blood sugar level can remain abnormally high. GTF contains the mineral chromium, the vitamin niacin (B3) and some amino acids. If you are lacking sufficient chromium, it is difficult for the cells to get the glucose they need and you will feel tired. You may then resort to eating something for energy, probably something sweet or made with white flour, and your blood sugar levels will rise further but, because these foods contain virtually no chromium or niacin, the problem will continue, you will continue to be tired, you may even become diabetic. Eating sugar is *not* the answer to your energy problems. Taking a chromium supplement may be.

7. Correct Biochemical Breakdown of the Macronutrients via the Metabolic Pathways within the Cell

Once the major nutrients, the fatty acids, amino acids and glucose have entered the cells, they have to be broken down. This has to happen via a sequence of well-constructed reactions, so that at various steps along the way some energy is 'shaved' off, used to recharge the flat battery (ADP) and convert it to ATP which can be carried away and used wherever energy is needed, as we described earlier. In the process the molecules break down, eventually, into carbon dioxide, water and, in the case of the amino acids, some ammonia.

There are various names for these pathways (the Embden-Meyerhoff pathway, the Krebs cycle, beta-oxidation of lipids, and so forth) but the details need not concern us here. Our concern is that the reactions should happen correctly, and for this to happen a variety of micronutrients have to be available. These include thiamine (vitamin B1), riboflavin (vitamin B2), niacin (vitamin B3), pantothenic acid (vitamin B5), pyridoxine (vitamin B6), vitamin B12, biotin, coenzyme Q10, magnesium, manganese, copper, iron and zinc (see Chapters Six and Seven). These are all important nutrients. They are nutrients that are lost, to a greater or lesser extent, when food is processed, when grains are milled and stripped of their bran and germ, and when foods are cooked. These nutrients are missing entirely from many 'foods' such as sugars, fats and alcohol. They are found in only low levels in fruits and vegetables that are picked before they are ripe, carted to depots and kept in storage. Since this covers most of the things that happen to the foods you eat before they reach your mouth, it is no wonder that you are often tired and lacking in energy.

8. Short-term Storage of the Energy Released, in High-energy Molecules

The short-term storage molecule for a manageable quanta of energy, as we have seen, is ATP. All the steps in its production involve the breakdown of molecules containing large quantities of energy, reducing them to small manageable units, like rechargeable batteries. The steps along the way require nutrients, mainly vitamins and minerals. Thus the generation and function of ATP is heavily dependent on a wide variety of micronutrients.

9. Ready Availability of these High-energy Compounds as needed

When the immediate supply of ATP is used up, more must be generated, even between meals. Some of this comes from the ability of the cells to draw in the glucose floating by in the bloodstream as part of your normal blood sugar level. This glucose can act as a quick source of energy and will be replaced later, either from your small stores of glycogen ('animal starch') stored in the liver or muscles, or from your next food intake.

Fats in the bloodstream can also act as intermediate energy sources, entering the cells and enabling them to top up their level of ATP. Again, this is a nutrient-dependent step, requiring, among other things, carnitine, methionine, lysine and vitamin B6.

10. Correct Storage and Release of Excess Energy in Long-term Energy Storage Molecules

When you eat more food than you need, one of two things can happen. In the case of fats, the fatty acids may simply be immediately built back up into triglycerides and stored in your fat deposits, your adipose tissue. These fat stores are in all the obvious and visible places like your abdomen, your buttocks, your thighs and so forth. Adipose tissue is also used to form a protective layer around your delicate internal organs. By forming a layer under your skin, it helps to keep you warm.

In the case of sugars and starches, the breakdown process starts and then, if you have eaten more than you need, these components are built back into larger molecules again; not back into glucose but into more fats. They too are then stored as part of your adipose tissues. As anyone who has tried to lose weight can tell you, this process of overeating and building up adipose tissue stores is all too easy.

Your adipose tissues provide structural protection, warmth and a storage depot for energy compounds that are available whenever you need energy but do not or cannot eat, either because you choose to diet or because food is not available. In primitive times when there were no food shops and no refrigerators (as today in areas of famine and food shortages), this ability to store 'food' within your own body saved millions of lives. Nowadays, in the affluent parts of the world, it is often seen as a disadvantage. Many patients tell me they would be perfectly happy if all the excess food they ate simply passed on through, avoiding the risk of gaining weight. The Romans had a way of doing this. At intervals during and after their feasts they went outside to vomit and so make room for more food. This may have provided an apparent short-term solution, but what it must have done to the inside of their oesophagus and stomach and the rest of their digestive system, quite apart from their health in general is dreadful to contemplate.

A further function of this adipose tissue has developed in modern times. Most of the toxins you eat are fat-soluble. This includes the various pesticides and food additives plus many of the pollutants you inhale. These fat-soluble substances travel with difficulty through the bloodstream unless they are attached to fats in the blood. Associated with the fats, they enter the adipose tissues and become stored there. This is fine in principal, but it means that when you use this adipose tissue for energy the stored toxins are released back into the bloodstream. They then pass through the brain and the rest of your body and can make you feel dreadful. It is possible that some people who have trouble losing weight do so because the body is reluctant to break down these fat stores thereby releasing the toxins. This suggestion is supported by the way some people have found that their weight gain, or their reduced ability to lose weight when dieting, followed a period when they were taking medical drugs or had consumed an increased load of toxins, such as after top-dressing in a local farm, or exposure to paint and varnish fumes, etc.

This isn't a book about weight loss, but it is worth commenting, as we shall when we cover Chronic Fatigue Syndrome, that the solution is to start with a detoxifying programme and then, and only then, to start on either the weight-loss programme or your energy programme.

Finally

From all this, you will see that it is not simply a question of 'getting away with' a junk-food snack when parents aren't looking, or eating whatever's around when you are too busy doing other things to consider what your body needs, or too tired to shop for, cook and eat a proper meal. You haven't got time *not* to do these things; you can't *afford* the energy loss of *not* doing them. If you don't chew your food properly, take care of your digestive system or ensure that you get an ample supply of all the required nutrients, you may well be tired, *very* tired. You may also find that your body runs out before the years do and you die young, exhausted or both. This need not happen, since the solution is relatively simple.

What To Do

- Improve your diet and supplement programme.
- Start one if you are not already taking supplements.
- Take digestive enzymes.
- Use aloe vera and slippery elm.
- Relax when you eat.
- Correct any problems in your mouth.
- Chew your food thoroughly.
- Eat sufficient fibre to have at least three soft and bulky bowel motions a day.
- Avoid allergens and toxins.

Go back though this chapter and mark any problem areas that you think may apply to you and commit to making the necessary changes. Here and throughout the rest of this book you will find many suggestions as to what you can do. Put these into practice as far as you feel they apply to you. If you feel you need further help, there are plenty of naturopaths and natural therapists well qualified to help.

Chapter Four

Physiological Aspects of your Appetite

Your Appetite Switch

Clearly an essential part of having sufficient energy is having and eating a sufficient quantity of food. Equally important is eating the correct quality of food. Since these two factors are important it would seem to be reasonable to look for a mechanism in the body by which you choose both the quantity and the quality of the food you eat. Unfortunately, what we find is not totally satisfactory.

There is indeed a mechanism that controls the quantity you eat: your appetite. Essentially, this is like a switch in the brain. When it is on you have the desire to eat, when it is off you don't. It is switched on until you have eaten sufficient quantity of food and then, when you are 'full', it turns off. You may still, of course, continue to eat, and probably will if something delectable is offered to you. Unfortunately, however, there isn't a mechanism in the body that steers you in the direction of the right quality of food. There isn't a method by which the cells can let the brain know which individual nutrients they need. In general, the choice of food is left to chance, whim, custom and availability.

This seems to have worked well in prehistoric times when processed foods weren't available and when it was easier to detect whether or not a food made you feel good. What I find with patients is that once they have given up all processed foods and are eating a diet approaching the caveman diet of Chapter Two, they are much more aware of what individual foods do to their bodies and how uncomfortable they feel when they eat processed foods high in calories from fats, sugars and refined carbohydrates such as white flour, and low in nutrients.

In Chapter One, we mentioned that, from the cell's point of view, the bloodstream flowing past it is a bit like a conveyor-belt smorgasbord, presenting to the cell all the 'food' that is on offer. I also mentioned that the big problem with this system, from the cell's point of view, is that the cell cannot put in an order if the specific substance it wants isn't there. If a cell, for instance, needs chromium or vitamin B3 and there is none going past, it simply has to do without. There is no channel to the brain to take the message up so that the brain can direct you to eat a food rich in these nutrients. When you eat, the cells in your body that wanted chromium and vitamin B3 can only hope you have chosen food wisely. If not, the best that can happen is that your appetite switch stays on, you eat something else, and perhaps this time the cells are lucky and you have chosen a food rich in the nutrients they need.

Sometimes the generalised complaints from all the cells in your body are so loud and so insistent that your appetite switch stays on and you go on eating long after you are 'full to bursting'. You have probably had the feeling of having eaten a big meal and yet you still feel like nibbling; you still want *something*, though you may not be sure exactly what it is you want, what it is that would make you feel satisfied. That is about as near as your body can get to telling you that you have consumed sufficient (or excessive) quantity, but inadequate *quality* of food and that some of the essential nutrients are still needed. Sadly, at this point, you have probably eaten your meal and so you take recourse to a second helping of dessert, a bar of chocolate or some other such low-nutrient food that certainly does not solve the problem. All this will do is add more to your fat stores and still leave you feeling undernourished, and probably tired.

I have had many patients who have insisted that they *had* to eat sugar: they needed it, their body craved it, even after a large meal. When I persuaded them to take a supplement of a strong B complex, they invariably reported that they no longer craved sugar.

A friend with whom I used to dine weekly used to help herself to a huge plate of food from the buffet, consisting of steak, chops, sausage and fried onions plus rice and pasta salads, and wonder how I could survive on the 'rabbit food' of my choice. Within weeks of taking not only B group vitamins but a full supplement of both vitamins and minerals, she ate less (steak only, the chop and sausage were abandoned) and different food (vegetable salads instead of the starchy ones). Not only did her health and energy improve, but she went from a size twenty-six to a size sixteen in five months without even trying to diet and with no call on her willpower.

This is one reason that anyone trying to lose weight should take a good, complete and strong vitamin and mineral supplement. Your adipose tissues store fat and energy but they do not store the micronutrients. When you are trying to lose weight you rely on these fat stores for energy and you have to make up for their lack of micronutrients somehow; otherwise your cells, via a variety of chemical reactions and nerve and hormonal messages to the brain, will scream that they are 'hungry' and you will almost certainly break your diet. It is much easier to lose weight if you are well nourished with all of the essential nutrients.

In addition to these metabolic appetite switches there are, of course, other factors that play a role in determining the amount you eat. Early social patterns are important. If you ate large meals as a child, you will continue to consider this 'normal' even if you *are* gaining weight. The size of your stomach is also important, since it is hard for someone with a small stomach to eat a large meal and more likely they will feel the need to snack between meals.

What To Do

In Chapter Two, I suggested that you should be grateful for, and make use of, the twentieth-century ability to make nutritional supplements to counteract the damage your present environment inflicts on you. The suggestion here is that you use twentieth-century knowledge of the nutrient content of foods to help you choose the best possible diet with regard to both quality and quantity. Your aim should be to avoid the malnutrition of overconsumption and under-nutrition. You need today's nutritional wisdom to avoid today's nutrient-poor food; food that is designed to tempt you into high consumption for yourself and means high profits for the manufacturers. Your health and your energy levels will bear witness to whether or not you have made the best choices.

Your Daily Metabolism

Your body goes through a daily cycle of events that can have a large role to play in the amount of energy you produce. Understanding some of these changes can help you to have more energy.

To understand the benefits of this cycle, we again have to go back to prehistoric times. Before we had the blessings of shops and the easy access to food that we have today, a major preoccupation of your waking life would have been food – getting enough of it for survival and using it wisely and economically. On waking in the morning, you would have needed energy, to hunt, to gather food, to run, to collect fuel and so forth. Thus it was important that at this time of day food was turned into expendable energy as efficiently as possible. By evening, you had probably either eaten while you were out gathering and hunting or, in more settled times, collected enough food to sit by a fire, cook it and relax. At this time you did not need a lot of physical energy. You did not want to waste the food you were eating by turning it into expendable energy that, since you were not physically active, would have been lost or wasted as you gave off body heat. At this time of day, it was more important that your body converted the food you ate into energy stores within your body, into adipose tissues, available for some time in the future when less food was immediately available but when you would need the energy.

To achieve these two different objectives, your body relied then – and still relies today – on a group of mechanisms involving hormones, nerves and other internal messages. *The food you eat early in the morning is turned into energy, the food you eat in the evening is turned into fat*. You have probably heard of the saying, 'Eat breakfast like a king, lunch like a knave and dinner like a pauper'. That is the way it should be if you want to get the maximum energy out of the food you eat. This is also why dieters are told to eat early in the day rather than late at night.

In a study of volunteers, one group was given 2000 calories of food a day and told they had to eat it all for breakfast. They were to eat nothing for the rest of the day. The other group was given the same food but told to eat it all for dinner and have nothing until dinner-time the next day. After six weeks, the two groups swapped and followed the other regime. The study was not aimed at weight loss but at seeing how the body handled food at different times of day. The results were interesting. When each group ate their food for breakfast, they lost an average of 1.6 lbs and had more energy. When each group ate their food for dinner they gained an average of 1.1 lbs and had less energy. Thus there was a 2.7 lb difference in the weight of the individuals and their energy levels went up over the twelve-week period when they changed their diet from dinner to breakfast. This has a message both for people who are trying to lose weight and for people who want more energy.

Unfortunately, this fits in poorly with our current social patterns, where the major family and social meal is dinner in the evening, but do what you can. At week-ends, for instance, make lunch the major meal and dinner a light one. If you live on your own and do not socialise a lot, it is easy for you to make the changes. If you can do nothing else, then make sure that even a three-course dinner is light on calories. A possible example would be consommé, followed by a salad and fruit for dessert. Then when breakfast comes around, tuck in to a more substantial meal.

Metabolic Pathway Switches

There is one simple pathway switch that has a lot to do with the amount of energy you need. Understanding the implications of this can encourage you to take the necessary steps to have more energy.

When you break down fats and carbohydrates, there is a sequence of reactions before they enter the Krebs Cycle. The latter can be thought of as a merry-go-round. There are several molecules in the middle, like the animals on their poles. The fats and carbohydrates, suitably prepared, enter this and, in spinning round, give off all their stored energy.

For this cycle to proceed, a lot of micronutrients are needed. Vitamin B1 is needed for carbohydrates to enter this cycle and a lack of it can lead to a sweet tooth. The other nutrients are mainly the rest of the B group vitamins plus several trace minerals. Now, this is where it gets interesting. If you have sufficient of these micronutrients, the cycle works smoothly: your food 'goes for a ride' and gives off its energy. If the micronutrients are not there, the food cannot enter the cycle. Instead, it turns round and is rebuilt into high-energy molecules and sent to the adipose tissues. In practical terms, this means that the lack of micronutrients diverts your food from turning into energy and sends it off to be stored as fat instead. This is not what you want if you are tired, nor is it what you want if you are trying to lose weight as well as have more energy.

Once again, we see how important these trace nutrients are. Make sure you get as much as you can from your diet and then top up with the appropriate supplements.

Chapter Five

Insufficient Macronutrients

In this chapter we will be considering the effect on your energy and your health of consuming inadequate amounts, or the wrong types, of macronutrients.

The macronutrients are the proteins, fats and carbohydrates that provide you with the raw material for the energy you need. Getting insufficient of these means you are simply not eating enough food. The answer is easy: eat more. If you eat too little, you will either burn up body fat to increase the number of calories available, or you will not produce all the energy you need. In our modern, westernised lifestyle, few people have insufficient food. Certainly it can happen, certainly some people in our society are starving, but by and large the problems of the so-called first world countries are the nutritional deficiencies of overconsumption and undernutrition. We eat too much and of the wrong foods. However there are some people who do eat too little, who are tired because they don't take in sufficient fuel. There are people who have to make an effort to eat sufficient quantities of food. There are a number of possible causes and most have solutions.

Poor Sense of Taste and Smell

You have a limited sense of taste, consisting of four sensations – sweet, sour, acid and bitter. Everything else – the flavours you 'taste' as the food goes down – is in fact smell. Be that as it may, if you have recently found your sense of taste diminishing, it could be a deficiency of vitamin A or zinc. You could be lacking in vitamin C. There are also some B vitamins that can damage your 'taste' buds (see Chapters Three and Six).

Mouth Problems and Dentures

If you need dentures, get them. If you have them and they don't fit perfectly, get them corrected. Eating is not an appealing activity if your mouth hurts or if the act of chewing causes you pain. People with dentures consistently make poor dietary choices, preferring soft and highly-processed foods to the high-fibre nutritious foods that would give them energy.

If your gums are sore or bleed, take Vitamin C and the bioflavonoids. Drink freshly-squeezed fruit and vegetable juices. Once your gums become less painful, eat a lot more raw fruit. As they become less painful still, eat salads. If your teeth have any cavities, are loose in their sockets or break easily, or if your nails have longitudinal ridges, increase you calcium intake, either from foods (mainly vegetables, not dairy products) or supplements. If, on the other hand, your nails have white spots, you probably need zinc; and if you have hang nails (those bits that can stick up at the sides), you may need manganese.

If you continue to have problems and cannot chew many foods, drink vegetable juices instead of eating salads. Make soups by lightly cooking the vegetables and then blending them. The soup will still be slightly chunky, but you will be able to swallow it without having to chew, and the vegetables will not be over-cooked. Make wholemeal flour into pancakes if bread is too difficult to chew. Mince meat, grind nuts. Do not be tempted to change to eating white bread and jam or other less nutritious and less energy-giving foods simply because your teeth and gums hurt. Above all, eat; do not let yourself become thin, tired and edgy.

Small Stomach

The textbooks would have you think that, inside, we are all the same. Far from it. Some people have small stomachs, others have stomachs twice or possibly three times as large as the stomach of another person. The person with a large stomach can eat two or three full-sized meals in a day. The person with a small stomach cannot. If you have a small stomach, you will eat as much as you can, feel full, and then be hungry long before the next mealtime. If you were brought up in a strict family where you were told to have three meals and no snacks in between you are probably slim and often hungry. If you have a small stomach, you should eat five or six small meals a day, but these meals should be of good quality. Do not make the mistake of assuming that the three 'in-between' meals are snacks and can be a few biscuits or a piece of cake. The quality must remain high if you want your energy level to be high.

If you are underweight, hungry and tired, try eating more often but reducing the total quantity each time. You will soon find out if a small stomach is a part of your problem or not.

Stress Associated with Meals

In some families, mealtime is the only time the whole family gets together. It was often the time Daddy was told of your misdemeanours, or you heard your parents arguing. If you grew up in this environment, mealtimes may have become associated in your mind with stress. As a result, you may either avoid eating or find that you are still tense at mealtimes. As a result, your digestion is impaired, as we have already discovered, and so your absorption of nutrients and ability to generate energy are diminished.

If this is the case, it is important that you make a special effort to relax before a meal: play calming music, think positive thoughts, do whatever it takes to make the necessary changes. Once you relax, your digestive juices will flow and you can then absorb your food and release the energy it contains.

Not Bothering

Some people do not eat enough because they are just too busy or preoccupied to think about it. They may not bother to shop; they may not bother to cook or prepare a meal. Either way, they will eventually be tired.

Look after your body. It's your home for this lifetime, and if it falls apart on you then you will not be able to do all those other things that seemed, at the time, to be more important than eating.

False Economies

Eating properly and looking after your body should be of paramount importance. Yet sometimes people put other things first. When money is short, they may buy clothes before food, or alcohol or cigarettes before food.

This is foolish. You cannot afford *not* to eat. It costs a lot of money to be sick. It costs a lot of money to be tired. You *lose* a lot of money when you are tired – too tired to walk so you have to take a taxi, too tired to work so your income decreases, too tired to take an interest in people and so you lose your friends. Invest in your nutrition, invest in your energy and your health, and you will have the ability to earn and achieve more, and you will avoid all the unwanted medical bills that can come about as a result of poor-quality nutrition.

Vanity

There is, in our society, a high value placed on being slim, sometimes on being slim to the point of absurdity. I have had several ballet dancers as patients, all trying to be slim to the point of emaciation and so not eating. They all wanted me to provide a diet that would give them much-needed energy and yet allow them to be thin as waifs. It seems they commonly live on bars of chocolate and cups of black coffee. This is no way to generate the energy they need and it is no wonder that they are so often tired. Models too try to eat sufficiently little to stay slim enough to disappear inside the clothes. Again, this is no way to have the energy they need for a physically demanding job.

Are you trying to be particularly slim? Do you spend days eating lettuce leaves and chicken wings and then feel tired and listless and so blow out on cakes and biscuits?

You can be very, very thin and yet still have lots and lots of energy, provided you have all the micronutrients you need to convert the food you do eat into energy rather than into adipose tissue. Ironically, it takes more B vitamins, for instance, to convert your food into energy than to turn it into fat. So get plenty of vitamins if you want to stay slim *and* energetic. The best way to do this is with the caveman diet described in Chapter Two, plus additional supplements. Make sure that you have sufficient macronutrients, particularly the proteins and complex carbohydrates, to deliver the energy you need. Be sure to avoid the sugars and saturated fats.

Anorexia

Anorexia is a physical and psychological problem and not one that we will consider here. My experience with people who are anorexic is that they live on nervous energy rather than normal energy. If they are bulimic as well, then they *are* eating the major foods, but since they vomit most of it back up they still do not get the energy they need.

There is a lot that can be done for both anorexia and bulimia but it is beyond the scope of this book. It almost always requires specialised help. It is a complex condition, usually resulting from a variety of emotional issues, although there may also be metabolic reasons for the problem.

I recall a patient of a colleague who, although tall and weighing only thirty-five kg (or about five stone), complained she was fat and wanted to know how she could eat less. She agreed to have a urinary amino acid test done and then take the appropriate amino acids as indicated by the results (she told us afterwards that she thought this would be a way she could eat less protein foods). Within three days, she phoned him in a panic, saying she was far too skinny, dangerously thin and demanding to know why no one had made her eat! We put this change down to an altered (and corrected) pattern of amino acid messenger molecules in her brain – a deficiency of one or more of them having, presumably, caused the altered perception that at thirty-five kg she was fat.

Types of Food

It takes a lot more energy to metabolise proteins than it does to metabolise fats or carbohydrates. Approximately five per cent of the calories that come from burning fats and carbohydrates for energy are needed to fuel the process of digesting, absorbing and transporting these fats and carbohydrates to the cells and then handling their combustion within the cells. On the other hand, it takes about thirty per cent of the energy you get from proteins to do the same thing. This is one reason why some people feel they can lose weight more easily on a high protein diet.

Using protein foods as a source of energy is highly inefficient. It also puts a strain on the liver and kidneys as they have to handle all the spare amine groups. These do not supply energy but rather demand it as they have to be carefully handled until they leave the body in the urine as dissolved urea and ammonia. Ideally, you should eat just enough protein foods to supply your protein and amino acid needs. This means consuming about twenty to forty grams of protein, but keep in mind that most protein-rich foods only contain around twenty-per-cent protein. Then build the diet up with carbo-hydrates until you have sufficient for your energy needs. Do not rely on protein for energy.

Chapter Six

Vitamins

Most of the vitamins are of vital necessity if you want to have sufficient energy. Many have some role to play in the process of generating energy, some of them have several roles to play. It is important that you understand these sufficiently, so that you become serious about getting adequate amounts of all of them.

It is not the intention here to go through a complete description of each vitamin. We shall simply be focusing attention on the specific attributes and functions of each vitamin as it applies to energy production and listing some of the symptoms you might have if you were lacking in that particular vitamin. Keep in mind, however, that the production of energy is a massive and concerted effort by the full range of metabolic processes within your body. You need them all, but the weakest link or links are the ones that need fixing most urgently and so a nutrient that may be the answer for you may not be the most important nutrient for someone else who is just as tired.

When we consider food sources of nutrients there are two approaches to take. You can consider which foods have the greatest amount of a nutrient on a per weight basis, for example per 100 g, or you can assess it on a per calorie basis. Since you (assuming your weight is constant) eat foods up to a total of your daily calorific requirement and not on the basis of the weight of the food, it makes good sense to pay attention to good nutrient sources on a per calorie basis rather than on the more usual per weight basis. In other words, consider the foods you eat on the basis of how many calories you have to consume to get your nutrient requirement. As an example, if you look at the table below, cabbage is clearly a better source of vitamin B3 than beef if you consider the calories you have to consume to get it.

	B3/100g	calories/100 g	B3/100 calories
Beef (rare)	4.5	260	1.73
Raw Cabbage	0.3	14	2.14

Where it is appropriate, sources of nutrients will be given on both a per weight basis and a per calorie basis. Where the lists would be similar, no distinction is made.

When considering deficiency signs, it is worth mentioning that several vitamin deficiencies can cause the same symptoms. For instance a lack of almost any B vitamin can cause fatigue. The more indications you have applying to one specific nutrient, the more likely it is that a deficiency of that nutrient is the culprit. It is not possible to rank the deficiency signs of any one nutrient in order of priority, as your body, other deficiencies and a variety of factors will dictate which tissues are affected first and most obviously by any specific problem.

Vitamin A (Retinol)

Vitamin A is not usually thought of as a vitamin that is involved in energy production. Its activity is more associated with the structures of the body, the bones and teeth, the skin and mucous membranes, and the myelin sheet around the nerves. It is also an important antioxidant and part of the immune system.

However, a long-term vitamin A deficiency has been found to lead to anaemia and it may have a role in the synthesis of haemoglobin. It is also associated with the metabolism of the thyroid hormones, T3 and T4, which are essential for energy management and which we will be discussing later (Chapter Ten).

Deficiency signs include
Problems with bones, teeth, hair, skin, mucous membranes and increased infections.

Sources include
Vitamin A: Liver
Carotene: Orange and dark green vegetables and fruits
N.B. beta-carotene is made of two vitamin A molecules, the other carotenes contain one.

Vitamin B Complex

As a group, the B vitamins are water-soluble and so readily transported in the blood. However, this also means they are lost if you throw out the water in which food has been cooked. They are also relatively unstable, being susceptible to light, heat, radiation, alkalis (like baking powder), light, UV and air. So if you keep food in bright light, cook it, leave it sitting around exposed to sunlight and then possibly reheat it, you will lose a significant amount of these vitamins.

Use wholemeal flour in cooking to get the B vitamins, but remember that you will lose some of the vitamins if you use baking powder. As an alternative to using baking powder when making cakes, you might like to think of using whipped egg whites and folding this into the mixture just before you put it in the oven. Even such small changes can make a significant difference to the amount of nutrients you receive from your diet.

Vitamin B1 (Thiamine)

Vitamin B1 is a key vitamin in the Krebs cycle, the one that converts sugars and fats into energy. Without it, this cycle cannot take place and you will have no energy, the food will be diverted to fat production instead. To a lesser extent, it is needed for the metabolism of some amino acids from proteins. If you have some thiamine but an insufficient amount, you will have some energy but not quite enough. This vitamin is critical for energy production.

It is needed by the nervous system as well as for the production of energy and this is a reason for many of the deficiency signs: they are essentially signs either of low energy or of a disturbance of the nervous system.

Deficiency signs include
Fatigue, and sleep disturbances.

Poor memory, decreased mental alertness, anxiety, irritability, confusion, headaches, depression.

Increased appetite, even when 'full' – particularly for sweet things, so use this vitamin generously if you are trying to get rid of your sweet tooth.

Numbness and tingling, burning sensations in the feet and toes, especially at night.

Stomach upsets, abdominal pain, constipation and sometimes diarrhoea.

Irregular heartbeat, palpitations and, in severe deficiency, worsening heart and breathing symptoms.

Painful calf muscles, muscle weakness and reduced reflexes.

The extreme B1 deficiency disease is beriberi.

Sources
Per weight basis: whole-grain products rather than refined or white, nuts, seeds and beans.

Per calorie basis: many vegetables (especially dark

green ones) are a richer source than grains on this basis.

Vitamin B2 (Riboflavin)

Vitamin B2 is also involved in the Krebs cycle – not so much at the start, as vitamin B1 is, but at several different steps around the cycle. So again, it is critically important for your production of energy. This vitamin is yellow and when you body has finished using it and the waste material is excreted in urine, it will make it more yellow. This is not a problem, nor does it mean that the vitamin hasn't been used thoroughly by the body before it was expelled.

You need thyroxin to convert this vitamin into its active form so if your thyroid gland is underfunctioning (see Chapter Ten), you may need additional amounts of this vitamin until you can stimulate your thyroid gland back into normal activity. You also need vitamin A for this, so again, although vitamin A is not usually thought of as an energy vitamin, in this indirect way it is important. Vitamin C protects vitamin B2.

Deficiency signs include
Depression, anxiety, worry, trembling, dizziness, lethargy and fatigue.
Seborrheic dermatitis with scaly and oily skin.
Red rims to the lower eye-lid, burning and itching eyes all made worse by bright light, eventually deterioration of eyesight.
Sore and burning mouth, cracked lips and cracks in the corners of the mouth, irregular surface to the tongue and painful swallowing.

Sources include
Per weight basis: whole-grain products rather than refined or white, meat, organ meats, milk, nuts and seeds.
Per calorie basis: vegetables such as watercress, leafy vegetables, broccoli, pumpkin, green beans.

Vitamin B3 (Niacin and Niacinamide)

Vitamin B3 is also needed for the Krebs cycle at several points around the circle. Without it, the cycle will slow down or even stop and you will have little or no energy. Unlike other vitamins, your body can make a certain amount of this one, provided you have an excess of tryptophan over and above your needs of this amino acid for protein formation and its specific functions. However, to get niacin from it you have to have some spare vitamin B2 and vitamin B6, which in any case is in high demand if you are on a high protein diet (one that would have spare tryptophan) and is also often in short supply. For this reason, it's usually much easier to make sure you get enough pre-formed vitamin B3 from your food.

Deficiency signs include
Anxiety, depression, irritability, fear, easily startled, poor memory and concentration, lack of initiative.
Weakness, debility, lethargy.
Muscle weakness, stiffening joints and tender joints and bones when pressure is applied.
Poor balance, burning or tingling sensations, fluid retention.
Dermatitis with redness, blisters, cracks, crusting, or shiny patches on areas exposed to sunlight, areas of friction, pressure points and areas exposed to body secretions.

Swollen shiny tongue, sore mouth, increased salivation with possible ulcers.
Bloating, flatulence, poor absorption, diarrhoea, blood in the stools.
The extreme B3 deficiency disease is pellagra.

Sources include
Per weight basis: whole grains, but don't rely on corn for the major grain in your diet, it is low in niacin and also in tryptophan. Other sources include organ meat, meat, poultry and fish.
Per calorie basis: most meats and some vegetables.

Vitamin B5 (Pantothenic acid)

Vitamin B5 is an essential part of the first step into the Krebs cycle. Without it, nothing can happen. By now you will have realised (a) how central and vital this Krebs cycle is to the production of energy, (b) just how important the various B vitamins are to its function and (c) the impossibility of having sufficient energy if you are short of the B group vitamins. Further, you will be realising how a lack of any of these vitamins can have a profound effect on your mood, behaviour and mental activity. The story continues with this vitamin.

Deficiency signs include
Apathy, fatigue, sleep disturbances, depression, irritability, impatience, aggression.
Headaches, altered skin pigmentation, stretch marks, acne and psoriasis.
Nausea, tooth-grinding, inflamed tongue, heartburn, flatulence, abdominal pains and cramps.
Burning feet and heels, shooting pains, muscle weakness, general burning or tingling feelings.
Adrenal exhaustion, erratic blood sugar levels.
Increased infections and palpitations.

Sources include
Per weight basis: organ meats, meats, egg yolks, whole grains and milk, nuts and seeds.
Per calorie basis: in general vegetables and organ meats surpass meats and grains.

Vitamin B6 (Pyridoxine)

Vitamin B6 is more important for protein metabolism than for the metabolism of fats and carbohydrates and so perhaps slightly less important for energy production than the others. However, we have already seen that it helps to generate vitamin B3 from any spare tryptophan you may have eaten. It also helps in the breakdown of stored body starch (glycogen) and the action of vitamin B5 on carbohydrate breakdown and energy production. It is involved in the metabolism of iron, a mineral that we shall see is essential for energy. Requirements are increased if you are taking the contraceptive pill.

Deficiency signs include
Insomnia, irritability, nervousness, depression.
Inflamed tongue and mouth.
Dermatitis, eczema and related skin problems.
Numbness and cramps, fluid retention.
Possible lack of dream recall.
Carpal tunnel syndrome – the tunnel that passes through the little bones of the wrist – includes pain and inflammation (pains like those of Repetitive Strain Injury).

Sources include
Per weight basis: whole grains, liver, nuts, seeds and beans.
Per calorie basis: vegetables and beans and lentils.

Vitamin B9 (Folic acid)

Unlike the B group vitamins above, all of which were involved in generating energy via the breakdown of sugars and fats, folic acid is important to the role of iron in the red blood cells. A lack of this vitamin can lead to anaemia (see Chapter Nine). Folic acid is also important for the formation of the genetic material, RNA and DNA and thus for the generation of new and healthy cells. A deficiency of this vitamin is relatively common, and it is one vitamin your doctor may actually prescribe. It is prescribed during pregnancy in recognition of its role in the correct multiplication of genes; although ironically, by the time you know you are pregnant, it is possibly too late since it is most important during the first minutes and days after conception occurs.

Deficiency signs include
Reduced number of red cells and so all the signs of anaemia (see Chapter Nine).
Reduced number of white cells and so increased risk of infections.
Poor healing of the skin and the mucosa such as the mouth and the lining of the digestive tract.
Restless legs, e.g. in bed at night.

Sources include
Per weight basis: corn bran, wheat germ, liver and a variety of vegetables.
Per calorie basis: just about all vegetables, particularly the dark green leaves.

Vitamin B12 (Cobalamin)

This vitamin is also essential for the role of iron in the red blood cells and a lack of it can also cause anaemia. It is an extremely large molecule and so somewhat difficult to absorb. To assist in the process, you produce a special carrier molecule called the Intrinsic Factor. Like hydrochloric acid, this Factor is secreted by the cells of the stomach walls; it then combines with the B12 and carries it along to the end of the small intestine where it also acts in facilitating its absorption into the bloodstream. It thus protects the vitamin, carries it through the small intestine and finally aids in the actual absorption. Conversely, a lack of Intrinsic Factor can lead to reduced transport, reduced protection and poor absorption of vitamin B12. Because of these potential difficulties it is possible that, even if you are getting sufficient in your diet, it may not be reaching the bloodstream and the bone marrow, where it is needed.

It is not easy to know whether or not you produce sufficient quantities of Intrinsic Factor, but since its secretion is related to the secretion of hydrochloric acid, you can look for insufficient acid as a guide. A minor lack of stomach acid may go undetected; a significant inadequacy can lead to a variety of digestive problems such as bloating, fullness and poor absorption of nutrients. So this may be provide a clue for you.

If, on the other hand, your digestive system is functioning normally, you benefit not only from the vitamin B12 you eat but also from the amount made by the normal and healthy micro-organisms in your intestinal tract. If you are a vegetarian and relying on this intestinally-synthesised B12, then a healthy digestive system is very important indeed. If your digestive system does deteriorate or you produce inadequate amounts of hydrochloric acid, as happens all too often, there is a further problem. Not only is absorption of B12 hindered and its synthesis reduced but a variety of unfriendly organisms, including yeasts that actually consume B12 are able to develop, thus rendering even the B12 in your diet unavailable. This same situation can also develop after you have taken antibiotics which in turn upset the normal flora. Later (Parts III and IV), we shall focus on the importance of a healthy digestive system in the treatment of health problems in general and Chronic Fatigue Syndrome in particular. This is just one of the many reasons why that is important.

A vitamin B12 deficiency can occur quite unexpectedly. This may be indistinguishable, at first glance, from a deficiency of folic acid, since both lead to anaemia. If folic acid on its own is given when the real problem is a lack of vitamin B12 the folic acid will resolve the anaemia but leave ongoing nerve damage caused by the lack of B12. This may not be detected until the damage is serious. For this reason, it is wise to take B12 whenever you are supplementing with folic acid.

Deficiency signs include
Those of anaemia including fatigue, apathy, pale skin, etc.
A deficiency has also been implicated in nerve damage leading to reduced motor and sensory function, poor co-ordination, muscle weakness and paralysis, stammering and even multiple sclerosis.

Sources include
The source of all vitamin B12 is micro-organisms, mainly those in the digestive tract of animals and humans. For this reason it is found more commonly in animal foods than in plants. Good sources include all types of meat and fish, eggs, and fermented products such as cheese, yoghurt and buttermilk.

If the problem is one of malabsorption of this vitamin rather than a dietary deficiency, then taking a supplement may not solve the problem. You may find you do better if you get an injection. Since it can be stored, mainly in the liver, one injection a month is usually sufficient.

Biotin (Vitamin H)

Biotin is not always thought of as a vitamin, although it was in the past called vitamin H. It is an important nutrient factor and is an essential coenzyme that works with enzymes involved in the metabolism of fats, carbohydrates and proteins and thus important for energy generation.

Deficiency signs include
Fatigue, irritability, depression.
A variety of skin and scalp problems, redness, eczema, dermatitis, and loss of hair and hair colour.
Sleep disturbances, nausea, altered tongue surface.
High cholesterol and atherosclerotic plaques.
Possible reproductive difficulties and birth defects and, according to some studies, SIDS (Sudden Infant Death Syndrome).

Sources include
Egg yolks, liver, brewers yeast, and the micro-organisms of the digestive tract. This latter is a major source. However, raw egg white contains a substance, avidin, that combines with biotin and blocks its absorption, so make sure you cook your eggs or you'll miss both the biotin in the yolks and the amount your micro-organisms are synthesising.

Choline and Inositol

Choline and inositol are nutrient factors commonly found as part of lecithin and important for the normal functioning of your liver and for proper fat metabolism. Choline is important for the production of adrenalin, which in turn stimulates target cells to generate energy on demand. It is also used for the synthesis of carnitine, the amino acid that assists fats into the cells so they can be 'burnt' and their energy released.

Choline deficiency signs include
Liver problems
Heart problems
Stomach ulcers
Kidney haemorrhage
Inositol deficiency signs include
Constipation
Eczema
Liver problems
High cholesterol
Sources of both include
Lecithin, egg yolks, soybeans

Vitamin C (Ascorbic Acid)

Vitamin C is important for the normal functioning of the adrenal glands and particularly in the metabolism of adrenaline and noradrenaline which are discussed later (Chapter Eleven). Without it, you would not be able to handle emergencies or maintain normal blood sugar levels (Chapter Fifteen). It is also important for the formation of other hormones in the adrenal gland including cortisone which also helps to provide energy and enable you to deal with stress.

Vitamin C is essential for the immune system. Without it, you are susceptible to all types of infections, from bacterial, viral and other sources. Even minor infections can deplete your energy level. Vitamin C is a natural antihistamine and so reduces the effects of allergies, many of which lead to exhaustion. It is needed for many reactions within the brain, often involving amino acids, that, when impaired, can lead to mood changes and altered levels of initiative, motivation and concentration, all factors associated with fatigue and lethargy.

It acts indirectly in many ways. It is needed for the activity of folic acid. It also helps to free iron from its carrier molecule, ferritin (see Chapter Seven). If this does not happen, you may be eating plenty of iron and it may be travelling around in your bloodstream, yet, since it is unavailable for the formation of haemoglobin, you may still be showing the signs of iron deficiency and anaemia. In that case, taking more iron is not the answer; it is more vitamin C that is needed. It has so many uses and functions, it is impossible to cover them all here. Suffice it to say that it is vital for your health, for your ability to handle stress and for energy production.

Deficiency signs include
Frequent infections.
Bleeding gums, easy bruising, broken capillaries, painful joints and muscles.
Decreased ability to handle stress.
The extreme Vitamin C deficiency disease is scurvy.

Sources include
Red capsicum, most fruits and above ground vegetables.

General

It is important to emphasise that there are other vitamins the body needs. There are even others that do have at least an indirect role to play in energy production. Many of the nutrients discussed above also perform many of the functions additional to those given. This chapter has been an attempt to describe for you the vitamins that are the most important for energy production and to highlight their role in this energy generation. It is by no means an attempt fully to describe each nutrient; far from it – that would take a book in itself.

What to Do

Diet: Make sure your diet is as good as you can possibly make it – and then improve it. I have had thousands of patients telling me they eat a good diet, that they have taken an interest in nutrition and that they eat sensibly and well. Then I look down at the dietary chart they have filled in and I am appalled, not only at what they eat but at what they consider to constitute a good diet.

> *I am reminded of a car-fanatic friend who had a beloved car that he worked on himself. Every weekend he could be found inside it, under it or over it, working on it. He thought he had it in absolutely perfect working order. One day he was stopped by a policeman who wanted to inspect his licence and give the car a quick look over. Without thinking, the man said 'No problem, look all you like, you won't find a thing wrong with this car.' This must have seemed like a challenge to the policeman, who immediately took a much more serious interest in it and found twenty-six points where it did not exactly comply with the regulations.*

No matter how good you think your diet is, it is almost certain that a professional could improve it for you. This is partly due to lack of knowledge – inevitable since nutrition, nutritional biochemistry and physiology are highly complex subjects. It is also difficult these days to keep up with the food technologists and find your way through the minefield of tricks the food manufacturers set up to convince you that the processed food they want to sell you is good, wholesome and nutritious. Depending on the country in which you live, 'wholemeal flour' may have lost as much as eighteen per cent of its content, almost all of which is the nutritious bran and germ. 'Wholemeal bread-making flour' may be only partially wholemeal and contain some white flour as well. 'Unsweetened' orange juice may have a permitted amount of sugar added ... And the list goes on. On top of that you almost certainly allow yourself a few cheats, thinking 'It will be all right, I eat well *most* of the time'. The trouble is, your body expects you to eat well *all* the time, and with the problems we encountered in Chapter Two that almost never happens, even when you *don't* cheat.

So work on your diet, improve it, and be watchful of the little slip-ups that start to creep in. Then take a general multivitamin supplement. If, after reading the above, you feel you have identified a particular nutrient that you need then you might want to take a specific supplement of it.

Supplements: You will have realised by now that the evidence points overwhelmingly to the need for supplements to boost your diet. If you identified specific needs from the lists of deficiency signs above, then eat the appropriate foods and take the appropriate supplements. If you felt that you needed them all, then take a good general-purpose multivitamin *and* a multimineral. Do not try to get them all in one tablet, they won't fit. If the label says it can provide all the nutrients you need in a single tablet, it is almost certainly underestimating your needs – or overestimating the size of the tablet it is possible for a human being to swallow.

When it comes to which type of supplements you should take, the problem can be tricky. I am often asked which brands I recommend and this is not easy, nor is the answer the same for everyone. Never doubt that in general cheap tablets are less good than the more expensive ones. They may contain only a small amount of each nutrient, or only a limited number of the nutrients, or they may not be well packaged into the tablet, in which case it is possible that some of the nutrients have been lost in the manufacture of the tablets or that you may not be able to absorb all the nutrients that are present as the tablet passes through your digestive system.

You should also realise that some of the individual nutrients, be they vitamins or minerals, are inexpensive, while some of them are costly. There is always a temptation for the manufacturer more interested in profit than nutrition, to load the mixture up with the less expensive ingredients. Sadly, the consumer will not be able to assess this as it is such a technical area.

I recall a time when I was acting as consultant to a company about to manufacture a range of supplements. I came up with a variety of formulations for them which they then costed. They pointed out that ingredient (a) was expensive and ingredient (b) was cheap, so if they decreased the quantity of (a) and increased the quantity of (b) they could market the product at a lower price. I pointed out that it would not work as well but this fell on deaf ears. Since then I have had a healthy scepticism about any product until I have used it on a number of people, including myself, and found one(s) that produced good results.

One good test is 'try it and see'. A good supplement should have you feeling better, no matter what your state of health. It should certainly help to improve your energy if you are tired, though it may not be sufficient to solve the problem if you are suffering from Chronic Fatigue Syndrome, for reasons we will discover later (Part IV).

The fact that someone you know felt better from taking a specific product is a help, though it is not a foolproof guide as their nutritional needs may be different from yours. However, if lots of people have benefited from different products of a specific brand you can start to trust that brand. Pick well-known and reputable brands, also ones that are sold in large quantities. People wouldn't keep rebuying them if they didn't feel the benefit. Do not pick the cheapest. While high price is not necessarily a sign of high quality, low price is almost certainly a sign of inadequate ingredients. If you do not experience the benefit, either change your brand or get professional advice.

REFERENCES

Roe, D.A., *Drug-Induced Nutritional Deficiencies*. The Avi Publishing Company Inc., 1976.

Chapter Seven

Minerals

Just as a number of vitamins are intimately related to your body's ability to generate energy from the foods you eat, so too is the activity of a variety of minerals important. We will consider them in this chapter. As with the vitamins, no attempt is made to cover all the minerals, nor all aspects of each one; instead we cover those with a significant role to play in the production of energy.

Before we start, there are several important differences between vitamins and minerals in the body that you should be aware if you are considering the possibility of deficiencies or of taking supplements.

Firstly, the vitamins are organic molecules that can be absorbed, used and excreted relatively easily by the body, with the possible exception of vitamin B12, which is a large molecule and so presents some problems, as we have seen. Minerals, on the other hand, are inorganic and are to a certain extent in a foreign environment when surrounded by all the organic molecules of the body. For this and related reasons, it is often more difficult to absorb minerals than vitamins, and for many of them to be satisfactorily absorbed a carrier molecule is necessary.

Secondly, it is quite appropriate to take a general multivitamin and let the body choose what it needs. With the minerals, on the other hand, since they tend to have specific carrier molecules to get them across the walls of the intestinal tract, and since many of the minerals, often in pairs, will compete for these carrier molecules, it is important not to upset any of the ratios. In this and other ways, if you take a mineral supplement that you don't need, you may aggravate a deficiency of one of the minerals that you do need.

Thirdly, whereas vitamins are made by the plant itself, minerals are obtained from the soil, which in turn gets them from the rock from which the soil was made and the ground water that passes through the soil. The plants absorb the minerals through their roots. If the minerals are in the rocks and soil in an available form, then some, at least, will travel up into the plant. If the mineral is not in the rock, soil or ground water, there is no way it can get into the plant. As we saw before, there is a further problem, (Chapter Two): If fertilisers and other chemicals used on the soil interfere with absorption, the minerals may not be available to the plant even if they *are* present in the soil. Once in the plant and in the food, however, the mineral stays there. Provided that when you cook it you consume the water or other liquid in which it was cooked, you will get the mineral; it cannot decay or break down as a vitamin might, since a mineral is an element and not a compound.

To abbreviate this, a plant makes vitamins largely independent of the quality of the soil, but once the plant is picked the vitamin content can decay. On the other hand, a plant cannot get or contain a mineral if it is not in the soil, but once it is in the plant it cannot break down.

What does this mean? It means that although you can read tables of figures giving the mineral content of foods, these are only averages and the particular food you eat may not contain the stated mineral content, and won't if that mineral was not in the soil, no matter what the books say. You may see that a certain food contains so much selenium. It probably does, when the plant from which it comes is grown on soil with a significant content of selenium. But if there is no selenium in the soil then it won't be in the plant. This makes it difficult to know just what quantity of the trace minerals you are getting in your food.

For all these reasons, it is desirable to test yourself and find out just which minerals you have in adequate amounts and in which you are deficient. Fortunately, a special test exists. Analysing a blood sample is not a good guide as the amount of a mineral in the serum or liquid of the blood is generally not indicative of the cell or tissue levels of the minerals. Analysing some tissue, such as the skin, would be painful and disfiguring. However, it has been found that analysing hair gives a useful indication of tissue levels. Hair Mineral Analysis has been done for many decades now and there is an accumulated pool of information on it.

By having a sample of hair analysed, you can get a lot of information, quickly and economically, not only as to your mineral levels but, via various mineral ratios, on the way different hormone systems, such as the thyroid (Chapter Ten) and adrenals (Chapter Eleven) are working. All this is extremely valuable when you are planning a supplement programme to give you more energy and improve your general health.

Now let's consider the individual elements and find out how they affect the production of energy.

Copper

Copper is one of the trace nutrients required by the body and plays a number of roles in energy production mainly related to the activity of iron, which is critical for the generation of energy, as we shall see shortly (in this chapter and in Chapter Nine). Copper improves the absorption, transport and incorporation of iron into hae-moglobin. It is also needed for the synthesis of haemo-globin. In these ways, it works with iron to help prevent anaemia and so maintain your energy levels by assisting the transport of oxygen through the blood and ensuring its delivery to the cells.

Within the cells, copper plays another role. It acts, again with iron, in the mitochondria – the powerhouses within the cells where the energy is generated.

Copper is needed independently of iron in the thyroid gland for the normal metabolism of the thyroid hor-mones. If these hormones are not produced in the proper amounts, you may have reduced thyroid activity and you will be tired (see Chapter Ten).

A deficiency of this mineral is unlikely if you are drinking or cooking with tap water from copper pipes. Otherwise, the possibility of a deficiency should be checked, preferably by Hair Mineral Analysis. It is also worth mentioning that, just as a deficiency can cause problems, so too can an excess. High levels of copper will cause toxicity signs. It will also compete with other minerals, such as molybdenum, for absorption and so could cause deficiencies of other minerals. It is important to take additional amounts only if you actually need them.

Deficiency signs include
Tiredness, anaemia, hypothyroidism.
Lack of skin pigmentation, altered appetite.

Toxicity signs include
Skin and nasal problems, bitter taste.
Mental disturbances such as hyperactivity and
schizophrenia.

Sources include
Drinking water if from copper pipes.
Carbonated drinks if passed through copper pipes
during processing.
Per weight basis: Oysters, liver, nuts, chocolate.
Per calorie basis: Oysters, liver, green leafy vegetables.

Chromium

Chromium is vitally important for managing your blood
sugar levels and for getting the glucose into the cells so
it can be used for energy. Without it, insulin cannot do
its job of pushing glucose into the cells, as mentioned
briefly earlier. This is how it works:

Whenever you eat sugars or starches, your blood sugar
level goes up. The pancreas then secretes the hormone
insulin. This travels through the blood and, essentially,
grabs hold of a glucose molecule and passes it across the
cell walls and into the cells. For it to do this successfully,
another molecule is needed, called Glucose Tolerance
Factor or GTF which consists of three amino acids, niacin
(vitamin B3) and chromium.

If you are short of chromium it is possible to have
glucose floating around in the blood stream and high
insulin levels, yet no glucose getting into the cells. As a
result you may be diabetic, your cells will not generate
energy efficiently and you will feel tired. Here again the
solution is not the seemingly obvious course. You need
chromium rather than the extra insulin you may be prescribed.

Deficiency signs include
Corneal lesions and opacity in the eyes.
Mood swings and lethargy.
Impaired glucose handling, high and erratic blood
sugar levels and glucose in the urine (if the deficiency
is severe).

Possible sources include
Per weight basis: brewers yeast, peanuts, prunes, clams,
corn, chicken, vegetables.
Per calorie basis: green leaves, tomato, mushroom,
vegetables in general.

Iodine

Iodine has one major role to play in the body; it is an
essential part of the thyroid hormones T3 and T4 (see
Chapter Ten). In fact, the numbers 3 and 4 in T3 and T4
refer to the number of iodine atoms in each molecule.
These hormones are made by the thyroid gland and it
is their secretion and action on target cells that determine
your metabolic rate, the rate at which your cells convert
foods into energy. This means that without iodine you
will be tired, run down, gain weight, feel the cold and
have no energy.

Two factors are important: both the consumption and
absorption of iodine and its incorporation into the hormone. The incorporation of iodine into thyroxin is
inhibited by a number of drugs and certain foods. The
foods concerned are the brassica family – that is, cab-
bages, cauliflower, broccoli, etc. – plus peanuts. This does
not mean that these foods will necessarily make you
tired, but they could be a contributing factor if you have
an iodine deficiency.

As is true for the other minerals or elements, iodine
can only occur in foods if it is in the soil. There are two

factors peculiar to iodine in regard to your food. It is more likely to be in the soil if you live near the ocean where salt-water spray is in the air, and it is commonly added to salt and since there is such an over consumption of salt, the incidence of iodine deficiency has been reduced.

Deficiency signs include
Lethargy, tiredness, feeling the cold and easy weight gain.
In more severe cases, goitre, with swelling of the neck and bulging of the eyes.

Sources include
Fish, dairy products, eggs.

Iron

The body contains a total of about 5g of iron, an amount that would easily fit on a teaspoon. Most of this – about a third – is attached to the protein molecule, haemoglobin, that occurs in red blood cells and gives them their colour. A small amount occurs in every cell of the body in the mitochondria, the cells' powerhouses where, ultimately, food is converted into energy. Another small amount is in the transport system, where it circulates continuously in the fluid of the blood (in addition to the iron in the red cells), ready to be delivered to cells that need it. The remainder, about a third of the total, is stored in the liver, the spleen and the bone marrow.

Iron is an interesting element, in that the body has no significant way to get rid of it other than by loss of blood. Other trace minerals can be lost in the urine whenever there is an excess in the body, but not iron. Perhaps it is too precious for the body to risk an easy deficiency in this way. Only a very tiny amount is lost in the urine and in the sweat; slightly more is lost via the liver and intestinal tract into the faeces. Even when combined, however, this amount is negligible.

Since it is not possible to get rid of an excess, there is a carefully-controlled mechanism in the walls of the small intestine that controls the amount of iron that is absorbed. If all works well, you will only absorb the amount you actually need.

Put simply, this is how the mechanism works. There is a molecule called apoferritin within the walls of the small intestine that is capable of picking up iron that passes through the digestive system. When it has collected as much iron as it can carry, it becomes iron-saturated and is called ferritin. Since the saturated ferritin cannot pick up any more iron, any other iron in the digestive tract will pass on down the line.

The iron-saturated ferritin then moves across to the other side of the mucosal wall, near the bloodstream. Here the iron is passed on to another protein molecule called transferrin. As soon as this has all the iron it can carry, it ignores any more iron attached to ferritin in the walls of the digestive tract and moves off, ready to deliver iron to whatever cells need it.

If no cells need iron, the transferrin remains saturated and continues to circulate in the blood. The ferritin in the walls of the digestive tract also remains saturated and any iron you consume will pass straight through. But when there are cells that do need iron, the transferrin will deliver it. It will then return to the walls of the small intestine and collect more from the ferritin. The ferritin, now unsaturated and hence called apoferritin, will return to the other side of the intestinal wall and pick up more iron from the food you have eaten.

That sounds fine, doesn't it? So how, given that you consume about 10 to 20mg a day and only need to absorb about 2mg, can you possibly become anaemic? There are many ways this can occur.

For a start, you need this seeming overkill as you are only able to absorb about ten per cent of the iron you consume. The iron in food exists in a variety of forms and complexes. Some of these release the iron for absorption more readily than others. Inorganic iron compounds in oxidised form, such as ferric oxide, ferric chloride or ferric sulphate, are poorly absorbed (so rust is of little use to you!). The reduced or ferrous form is better absorbed. Organic compounds, such as iron chelates, ferrous citrate, ferrous ascorbate, ferrous gluconate, are absorbed slightly more readily.

The most easily absorbed form of iron, however, is that already combined with haemoglobin in the blood of other animals and therefore obtained from meat. There is iron present in other foods, in vegetables and whole grains, but it is much less well absorbed. Much of this iron is present in the oxidised ferric form, which has to be reduced to the more desirable and more soluble ferrous form in the stomach with the aid of the hydrochloric acid there. If you are producing inadequate amounts of hydrochloric acid in the stomach, and many people are (particularly people who are over thirty or into their forties and beyond), then this step may not happen efficiently. As a consequence you are likely to absorb less iron from your food. Think back to what was said about this in Chapter Three. By now you should be realising just how important your stomach acid is and the great number of problems a deficiency can cause.

A number of factors improve the potential iron-absorption efficiency. One of these is vitamin C. It improves the conversion of ferric iron to ferrous iron; it chelates or combines with the iron, thus converting it into a readily absorbed form; and, in the acid form, it makes the stomach contents slightly more acidic. In fact, vitamin C can be so successful at this that it can even help the iron to bypass the ferritin–transferritin route.

This is rarely a problem, particularly in women who menstruate each month, but in men who suffer from a rare disease involving excessive iron absorption, this factor should be considered. If you do take an iron supplement in an unchelated form, such as ferrous sulphate, combine it with a protein-rich food to increase its absorption efficiency.

One problem that can occur when you take an iron supplement, particularly as ferrous sulphate, is constipation. If this happens, then switch to an organic or chelated form of iron rather than the more common ferrous sulphate usually dispensed by doctors and pharmacists.

Deficiency signs include

Pallor. Iron, as part of haemoglobin, is responsible for the red appearance of your tissues. Therefore when you look unusually pale you may well be short of iron. So some of the easiest signs of iron deficiency to detect relate to this.

Look for a lack of the usual red coloration inside the lower eyelid Your nails can give you lots of clues. Is the nail bed pale in colour? Does it stay pale for longer than usual when you first press it and then release the pressure? If you are not sure, check your own nails against someone else's when you do this. If the nails themselves are flat or even concave, this is another clue. Your hands can help as well. Stretch them out with the fingers as far back as possible and observe the lines crossing your palm. They should be bright red; if they are pale, anaemia may be part of your problem.

Other signs: You can be lacking in iron and yet not be anaemic. Other iron deficiency symptoms include a sore, flat or shiny tongue, possibly with cracks on the edges, mouth sores and cracks at the corners and difficulty swallowing.

Sources include
On a per weight basis: bran, spirulina, molasses, liver, pistachios, sunflower seeds, oysters, parsley, heart.
On a per calorie basis: parsley, chard, spirulina, oysters, sauerkraut, molasses, vegetables, liver, heart.

Magnesium

With this mineral, we are back to the Krebs cycle, that crucial sequence of reactions in the production of energy. Magnesium is another essential nutrient in this cycle and without it you will not have sufficient energy. We mentioned earlier the high-energy molecule, ATP, which acts like a short-term battery in the storage of tiny amounts of energy and which can provide this energy at a moment's notice when and where it is required. Magnesium is essential for ATP to do its work. Magnesium is also involved, with vitamin B6, in protein metabolism and the building of strong muscles. A lack of magnesium can put your nerves on edge and upset your heart.

Deficiency signs include
Weakness and lethargy, mental disturbances.
Muscle cramps, hiccups, convulsions, vertigo.

Sources include
On a per weight basis: seeds, whole grains (75% is lost during conversion to white flour), nuts.
On a per calorie basis: vegetables.

Manganese

This mineral is often lacking in the diet. Of over two hundred patients I tested in a study in Australia, approximately eighty-five per cent were manganese-deficient. This and chromium (at eighty-three per cent) were the two minerals most commonly lacking.

Its absorption is hindered by calcium, phosphorous, iron, cobalt and zinc. It is therefore possible that if you are busily supplementing with calcium in an effort to avoid getting osteoporosis, iron because you have heard it is good for energy, and zinc because you have read about it and have white spots on your finger nails, you may be creating a manganese deficiency. Here again, it is obvious that you should check your levels before planning a mineral supplement programme.

Manganese is essential for bones, joints and other connective tissues and it is possible that many a structural pain could be avoided if the amount of manganese was increased. As far as energy production is concerned, it effectively helps to draw glucose into the cells, by encouraging compounds that help the Krebs cycle to function and it is also used at many points along the pathway of converting carbohydrates into energy.

Like other minerals, having too much can also cause problems. It is rare to consume an excess of manganese, but if you do it may interfere with iron metabolism and cause anaemia.

Deficiency signs include
Mainly symptoms to do with joint, bone and muscle pains, from clicking, cracking or creaking joints to outright aches.
Nail problems, including 'hang nails', the bits that can stick up along the sides between the nail and the skin.

Sources include
On a per weight basis: whole grains (about 98% is lost in converting it into white flour), nuts and seeds.
On a per calorie basis: vegetables.

Zinc

Zinc works with at least eighty different enzymes in facilitating a wide variety of reactions throughout the body – many of them involved, both directly and indirectly, in the production of energy. It is also needed for the production of insulin, the hormone that drives blood glucose into the cells so that it can be available for energy production.

Deficiency signs include
Lethargy, lack of energy, mental confusion and/or hyperactivity.

Sources include
On a per weight basis: bran, wheat germ, oysters, seeds, nuts, meat.
On a per calorie basis: oysters, endive, seaweed, meat, parsley, clams, shrimps.

General

Keep in mind that no attempt has been made here to give a complete picture of what each mineral does in the body, nor to cover its actions in detail. That discussion is reserved for a book on overall nutrition. The focus has been on the minerals that are most important for the production of energy, the way they are involved in the production of energy and what happens if you are deficient in that mineral. Finally, it is worth emphasising that, if you think you have mineral deficiencies, it is well worth the effort of finding out, before you take supplements of only one or two. Fortunately the test, Hair Mineral Analysis, is easy, painless and relatively inexpensive. Any natural therapists should be able to help you to get this done.

Chapter Eight

Your Energy, Your Environment and Toxins

We have already alluded to the fact that toxins can cause or contribute to your health and energy problems, and we shall now consider this topic further.

Many substances harm your body. In addition to generating their own specific symptoms, they frequently reduce your ability to produce energy, or increase your need for energy. They may be toxic elements like lead or chlorine; they may be molecules such as drugs, agricultural and food additives or other pollutants; they may be organisms, such as *candida albicans*, and the toxins they produce; they may be viruses or bacteria; or they may include such things as radiation, cathode rays, X-rays and so forth. In other words, the term 'toxins' encompasses many things, physical or chemical, atoms or molecules, living or dead; all of which have a negative impact on your body and energy levels, making or keeping you tired and unwell.

In this chapter, we shall be looking ahead somewhat, since toxins can have an impact at two levels. Firstly, at a mild level and while you are relatively healthy but tired (though not totally exhausted), they will have their specific toxic effect. This will be essentially the same effect for everyone. Secondly, once your total toxic load has become excessive, and your immune system and general health sufficiently depleted as a result, you will develop generalised systemic symptoms of an overall toxic overload. This is an inherent part of Chronic Fatigue Syndrome, when you become acutely and uniquely sensitive to the toxins in a way not experienced by less unhealthy people. This is how it works:

Environmental and Food Toxins

I recall hearing of a woman who had moved into a large caravan to live. The walls of the van, the cupboard doors, etc. had been treated with formaldehyde. Living in it, exposed to the fumes night and day, had lead to an overload and she had become acutely sensitive to them. She had to move into a new home. Soon after that, she entered a room and was talking to a man who, unbeknownst to her, had a cigarette in the hand behind his back. Within minutes she had reacted and passed out cold on the floor. When the problem was identified and the cause recognised, she was amazed, saying that cigarette smoke had not bothered her before. It hadn't, but now that she was over-sensitised to the formaldehyde in it (by the fumes in her home), even the smallest amount was capable of producing severe symptoms.

Keep this double aspect of toxins in mind as you read this chapter, and beyond. There is the overt damage a substance may cause to people in general, which you and others will recognise. There is also the possibility of your own idiosyncratic (and possibly recently developed) acute sensitivity. It may have come about as a result of over-exposure. It may have come about as a result of even a small or normal exposure when you were unwell, and exposed to a variety of chemicals all at once. You may have been exposed to physical hazards such as radiation; you may have been particularly under-nourished following a period of bingeing on junk food or alcohol or giving up on your supplement programme. Many different factors could have led to the problem.

The list of possible toxins we could consider is endless, so no attempt will be made to be complete. Rather, it is intended that you should begin to get an understanding of what toxins can do to you and the relative importance to your health of either dealing with them or avoiding them. So much of what we are led to believe is safe can in fact cause problems.

It is virtually impossible to live in the twentieth century without being exposed to a wide range of toxins. Even if you live in some remote part of the Himalayas or central Africa, or the centre of the Antarctic, you will be exposed to a variety of man-made or man-induced hazards, from an individual substance which you might ingest to the global effect of changes in the ozone layer. Do not let the list, overwhelm you. The sensible plan is to do all you can to avoid as many toxins as possible without making life intolerable. Then nourish your body with the best possible diet and supplements and trust your immune system to protect you from the rest. You don't, for instance, have to breath in hair-spray; you can open windows when you are using cleaners, etc. You can control the food you eat at home. Avoid the majority of agriculture chemicals by buying organically-grown food and unprocessed foods; trust to your immune system when you eat out. Avoid food stored in plastic, served in plastic or Styrofoam (particularly hot food and drink), or eaten with plastic utensils. Even the lining of tins and cardboard food cartons can cause problems.

Your home environment can be lethal, often with a higher level of toxins than anywhere else. It all depends on how many oven-sprays, ironing-sprays, cleaning solutions, disinfectants, deodorisers, glues, perfumes, polishes, hair-sprays, detergents, bleaches, insect killers, dry-cleaning fluids, window cleaners and so forth, you use, and the amount of plywood, particle board, plastic, artificial carpets and other treated materials and fabrics you have. If you can smell something, that means some of the substance has reached your smell sensors at the back of your nose: you have taken whatever it is into your body. If you were to list the ingredients of even one of these sprays or substances, along with a description of the possible harm each ingredient might do, you'd almost certainly throw the lot out right away. Think of what hair-spray does to your hair. Do you really want hair-spray lining your lungs? The chemicals in the spray-packs that damage the atmosphere are blown into the air you breathe. Even if you use a non-aerosol spray, the chemical effect on *you* can be disastrous. Smell is no absolute criterion. There are molecules in the air that can harm you but have no smell. Think of the classic suicide method: a hose from the car exhaust pipe plumbed into the window of an otherwise sealed car. Carbon monoxide has no smell.

The home problem is exacerbated if you seal it up tight, run air-conditioners and/or central heating and have a television going.

Plastic materials degas. A few molecules are constantly flying away, moving through the air and probably entering your lungs. Think of the atmosphere when you get into a new car; you can smell the leather or plastic. You are taking these molecules into your body. The leather may not be too bad as it is of animal origin and can probably be metabolised, but you should still be wary of chemicals used in treating it and other fabrics. The Mad Hatter was no figment of Lewis Carroll's imagination: hatters are exposed to dangerous toxins. Plastics are worse than leather. Be careful about home-decorating: you are bathed in an atmosphere of chemicals, even after the smell has gone.

Your office is often worse than your home, if it is a huge building and is sealed and air-conditioned. Add fluorescent lights, photocopier chemicals, printer inks, whiteboard markers and acres of degassing plastics. The chemical and physical hazards at work can be so bad, particularly in large buildings, that the problem is now thought of as a specific entity, a workplace hazard, and labelled 'Toxic Building Syndrome'.

In your ordinary daily life you could be exposed to any number of toxins and it is rarely possible to pick the main culprit. It is difficult to say, 'I have these three symptoms, so I must have been exposed to XYZ, I will locate its source and avoid or eliminate it.' It doesn't happen like that. Many of these substances cause a range of similar or overlapping symptoms. They often act on the nervous system and so cause headaches, confusion, dizziness, lethargy, lack of initiative, tiredness, exhaustion, anxiety, nervousness, weeping and depression and multiple mood changes. You may feel tingling or numbness, get muscle cramps, be short of breath or find that, as a result of a weakened immune system, you are getting frequent colds and other infections. You may also be exhausted.

This is a confusing conglomeration of symptoms for the average doctor or practitioner not well versed in the effect of environmental toxins. If your doctor has not been able to find a specific illness to which your symptoms can be attributed, they may have told you (or at least implied) that it is 'all in your head'. This is usually taken to mean that you are imagining things, or that your symptoms are the result of your current worries and anxieties. However, 'in your mind' can have another meaning – namely, 'in your brain'. The majority of chemical toxins have at least some, and often a major,

effect on the brain and its chemistry. You already know
what alcohol, marihuana, cocaine and other drugs, even
coffee, often in tiny amounts, can do to your brain. Thousands of other substances, freely permitted to be used
and spread through the atmosphere and in our food, can
have much the same effect.

One of the reasons why these chemicals so often affect
the brain is that many of them are fat-soluble. Think
about it: if they were water-soluble, they would be
washed away. Water-soluble pesticides, for instance,
when sprayed onto crops, would be washed off in the
first rain. Oil-soluble ones, on the other hand, remain as
an oil film around the fruit. Many of the toxic chemicals
are derived from the petro-chemical industry and are
organic molecules soluble in fats, including the fatty
parts of the body.

This has two effects. Firstly, your brain, as an organ,
is rich in fats, so a high proportion of the chemicals to
which you are exposed can lodge within the fats in
your brain. The interconnecting nerve cells are intimately
interwoven with and surrounded by a complex collection of lipids or fats, many of them with specific roles to
play in the normal functioning of your brain. Many of
the toxins can become concentrated in the nervous
system and cause local damage.

There is a second problem. You will recall that whenever you eat more than you need, be it fats, carbohydrates or proteins, the excess is converted into fats
and stored in your fat deposits or adipose tissue. This
then becomes a readily-available storage centre for all
these fat-soluble toxins. All is well while your weight
remains constant or increases. Problems start, however,
when you go on a diet and try to lose weight. As soon
as these, possibly toxin-laden, fat deposits start to break
down, the toxins are released and enter the bloodstream.
In time, this blood flows through the brain. The chemi-

cals will either effect the brain directly by reacting on the nerve cells, or become absorbed into the fats of the brain. The resulting symptoms can put you off dieting forever. If you find that when you go without food for a while (and so release stored fat for energy), go on a fast, a cleansing programme (such as eating only fruit and vegetables), or a diet, you feel dreadful, this may be the cause. This does not mean you should give up the cleansing programme or diet. It does mean that you have some work to do. You may have to hasten slowly; but the worse the symptoms are, the more important it is that you get rid of the toxins.

All these toxins put a strain on the body and use up energy reserves. Dealing with them can leave you not only with a variety of symptoms, but feeling tired and lethargic.

Your Body's Detox Mechanisms

You have several ways of getting rid of toxins. Minor ways include via exhaled air; via mucous such as from your lungs, nose and vagina; and via the skin, both through the pores in sweat and in the cells as dead cells fall off. The two major routes that will concern us here are via the kidneys in the urine and via the liver and digestive system in the stools.

Most readily-soluble toxic substances move relatively freely round the body in the bloodstream. They may be taken into cells where they are broken down into smaller and (hopefully) safer molecules, which in turn are passed back out into the bloodstream. Whether they have been worked on by the cells or not, they eventually pass through the kidneys which let them through the filtration system and they leave the body in the urine.

If you are fortunate, this conversion has created compounds less dangerous than the original substances.

Sometimes, however, the body makes a mistake and a more dangerous compound is made. Alcohol, mildly harmful to the body itself, is converted into acetaldehyde and epoxides which cause problems of their own, in addition to and sometimes worse than those caused by the alcohol from which they were made. Some compounds from cigarette smoke are converted into even nastier compounds in the blood. Nitrates in food are converted to the more dangerous nitrosamines in the stomach after reaction with the amino acids of proteins.

As an aside, it is worth pointing out that this is why some manufacturers claim that their products are harmless. They may well be harmless, but their by-products within the body can be very harmful indeed, even to the point of causing cancer as in the case of nitrosamines.

Either way, if the toxin load is high or particularly toxic, damage can be done to the kidneys and the exit tubes including the bladder. In time, this can result in a variety of symptoms, including exhaustion; symptoms which are new and may leave you complaining that so-and-so can't be the problem since you have been coping with it all your life: it can't suddenly be causing kidney or bladder problems, nausea, headaches and confusion. It can't suddenly be making you tired . . . It can. It is a case of overload, or the last straw (see Chapter Eighteen).

Less soluble substances, substances that are fat-soluble rather than water-soluble, fats and some more dangerous toxins, are dealt with differently. In some cases, they too are metabolised, at least partially, by the cells, usually but not always to less harmful compounds. In other instances, the substance may remain intact. Either way, what is left and cannot be lost via the urine remains to be dealt with. It is common to find that a protective carrier molecule, often an amino acid or protein, is attached to the toxin. This usually reduces the damage it can do. The fat-soluble toxins also travel through the bloodstream as part of the lipoproteins we shall discuss in Chapter Nineteen, particularly the low-density ones. The protein complexes then pass through the liver, along the bile duct, into the intestinal tract, on to the colon and out in the stool. The lipoproteins are also worked on in the liver and some of their toxic load may also be discharged via the bile duct. If you are unlucky, some of the toxins released into the intestines in this way may be reabsorbed, but at least you will have lost some, and the cycle can be repeated.

There is commonly a limit to the quantity of toxins you can deal with in this way, a limit to the amount of protective carrier compounds the body can make and a limit to the load the lipoproteins can handle. In part, this limit is dependent on the activity of enzymes, which in turn is dependent on the amount of cofactors present, the amount of vitamins and minerals. For this reason, on a detox programme you will almost certainly be told to increase your nutrient intake considerably. (See Chapter Twenty-Seven.)

If you are loading the body with more toxins than it can handle, they accumulate and can continue to cause problems long after you have taken them. Patients often ask me how long it will be before they feel a result from taking supplements. You may be asking the same. How long is a piece of string? It depends on whether or not your detox system was overloaded and has a backlog to deal with. It depends on whether or not you continue to take in either toxins or substances to which you are allergic or acutely sensitive. It depends on your general state of health and the amount of damage that has already been done, to the mitochondria, or to the liver, kidneys and the other organs that have suffered in the fallout. It also depends on how thoroughly you follow any treatment you start. If you would like to know what

to do if you want to put your own body through a detox
programme refer to Chapter Twenty-seven.

All these reactions require energy and leave you with
less energy for other purposes. In addition, since the
reactions within the cells may damage the mitochondria,
the units in which most of the reactions occur while
converting glucose and fats to energy, your energy production capacity can be significantly reduced.

Toxins in the Digestive Tract

A wide variety of toxins either travel through or orig-
inate in the digestive tract. Here, they and you are susceptible to the health and integrity of this tract in general
and to the types of micro-organisms that are present in
particular. Many types of micro-organism can have an
adverse affect on the integrity of your digestive tract,
including parasites, moulds, fungi and bacteria.

By their presence, these organisms already indicate a
local problem. If your digestive tract was healthy, these
organisms would not be able to get a foot-hold. This
local problem means that your normal digestion and
absorption of food and nutrients is compromised and we
have already seen how your energy levels can fall as a
result. Secondly, the organisms will do their own
damage: they interfere with the nutrients you have consumed, either damaging them, impeding their absorption into your system or absorbing them themselves.
Thirdly, if harmful bacteria or moulds are present, then
the normal healthy bacteria that you need and want
are almost certainly absent. Many of these beneficial
organisms make valuable nutrients for you, such as
biotin, vitamin B 12 and several other B vitamins, plus
vitamin K. Fourthly, the organisms almost certainly produce a variety of chemicals that are harmful to you.
Candida albicans is a good example of this, producing

a number of toxins that contribute to the symptoms of candidiasis, as we shall see shortly (Chapter Sixteen).

Organisms, particularly moulds and fungi, can cause serious damage to the lining of the digestive tract. They can decrease your absorption of nutrients where this requires specific carrier molecules (see Chapter Seven). They can also facilitate the absorption of unwanted toxins and of food particles that have not been properly digested. This latter effect may contribute to chemical sensitivities and food allergy problems that in turn can make you tired.

There is a simple urinary indican test that can be done to determine the level of bowel toxins, but in essence, if you get at all bloated or pass wind, if you don't have three regular bowel movements a day and if you are not totally healthy, then the problem of toxins and your energy could well start here in the digestive tract. This is why you will find that most programmes designed to help you increase your energy will focus on some sort of detoxification programme combination with steps designed to improve the function of your digestive tract, as well as focusing on the supply of nutrients. This is particularly true for serious fatigue as in Chronic Fatigue Syndrome or CFS which we will be considering later (Part IV).

It is now time to look at a few specific toxins. This is by no means a complete list. A complete list of the toxins within our environment with explanations of what they could do to you emotionally and physically would fill a large book. They are, however, examples of some of the relatively common toxins. This section is also designed to alert you to a situation you may have been trying to ignore or of which you may have been unaware.

Toxic Elements

Chlorine, as found in drinking water and in swimming-pools, is a strong oxidising agent and greatly increases your need for all nutrients, particularly the antioxidants such as vitamin A, C and E and the minerals magnesium, manganese, copper and zinc. If you don't supplement, a deficiency of these nutrients can cause tiredness, in addition to the other damaging effects of chlorine. Fluoride increases your need for magnesium and can cause a wide variety of other symptoms.

Minerals

Many of the minerals or metals are toxic and can cause problems. They all stretch your body's overall capacity to get rid of toxins and they all deplete your energy reserves. Even minerals that are essential for life in small amounts can, if you are exposed to major overloads, cause toxic problems.

Copper, for instance, is an essential nutrient. Without it, you would be anaemic and your cells would not be able to process glucose or fats for energy. High doses, however, have been known to cause hyperactivity in children, reduced ability to concentrate, irritability, postpartum depression and even schizophrenia. Other symptoms include arthritis, eczema, nasal irritation and a bitter taste in the mouth. The answer is to reduce your exposure to copper by drinking and cooking with purified water that has both passed through a reverse osmosis membrane and been filtered, and avoiding other sources, which include insecticides, beer, vinegar and carbonated drinks if they have passed through copper pipes, milk and copper cookware. Take extra zinc to balance out the copper.

Manganese is essential for a number of reactions

related to energy and the connective tissues. In excessive amounts, however, as you may experience if you are under the fallout from jet engines, it can cause neurological and respiratory problems.

Aluminium is not an essential nutrient and is only known for the harm it can do if you ingest or absorb it. It is obtained mainly from aluminium saucepans, frying-pans, teapots and kettles and from other aluminium kitchen utensils, aluminium foil and aluminium cans. It is also found in beer, milk, free-flowing salt, baking powder, pickles and maraschino cherries. It occurs in many deodorants, so look for one that is aluminium-free. It is a component of the usual medically prescribed antacids. It is an environmental pollutant from industrial waste, car exhausts, pesticides and cigarette filters. It can have profoundly harmful effects. It is found in the brains of people with senile dementia and Alzheimer's disease and is thought to cause senility and loss of memory. In the digestive tract, it can cause inflammation, burping, flatulence and even colitis. It also binds with phosphate and may cause osteoporosis and painful muscles. You can get a skin rash from the deodorants, and aluminium can cause kidney and liver damage. In children, it has been linked with hyperactivity and psychosis.

Arsenic, a well-known poison, is found in insecticides and pesticides, and so can be in anything you eat and drink unless you stick to organically grown produce. It is also an industrial pollutant, occurs in coloured chalk, car exhausts and in some paints. Any reader of detective stories will tell you that arsenic can be lethal and is often obtained as a rat poison. Symptoms include headaches, confusion and sleepiness. You may feel weak, experience burning pains, swelling of feet and hands, and get dermatitis, especially around hair roots. Your breath may smell of garlic and you may have a garlic taste in your mouth.

Cadmium is found in drinking water that has passed through galvanised iron pipes and in soft drinks from vending machines. It is in flour (white or wholemeal), but in wholemeal (and not in white) flour, there is zinc in the bran to balance the cadmium. It is in many processed foods: evaporated milk, oysters, kidney, liver, cigarette smoke, superphosphate fertilisers, silver polish and many industrial pollutants, pesticides, rubber tyres, burning motor oil, plastic, batteries, etc. High levels can cause fatigue directly, as well as the fatigue that comes as a secondary effect from all the other symptoms. It can increase your blood pressure, cause anaemia, diminish your sense of smell and damage your lungs. Your liver may be damaged, your bones may be painful, and you may get arthritis. Cadmium can affect your liver and kidneys, may be carcinogenic and can be lethal.

Lead, as we all know by now, is present in the petrol fumes that spew into the atmosphere daily. Many people living, working or going to school on or near busy main roads have shown high hair lead levels. There are many other industrial sources of atmospheric lead. Lead can also enter the food chain if plants are grown near the roads. Cigarette ash, car batteries, some mascara, some painted pottery and glass and some canned foods contain lead. Symptoms of lead toxicity include hyperactivity and learning difficulties in children. As an adult, you may experience headaches, dizziness, insomnia, depression, nervousness, irritability, anxiety, confusion. You may have weak and sore muscle and joints, or gout. A variety of digestive problems can occur, including loss of appetite, abdominal pain and constipation. Fatigue is probably a consequence of impaired adrenal function and induced iron deficiency anaemia. If you are exposed to lead, you should increase your intake of zinc which competes with it. By increasing your intake of calcium, you make sure there are less calcium 'holes', or positions in the bone into which the lead can slot, since it is the same shape and size. You are also more at risk to lead if you are iron-deficient, so make sure you are getting sufficient iron.

Then there is mercury. The most common sources of mercury include dental amalgams and fish from mercury-polluted waters. Don't play with liquid mercury if your thermometer breaks, even though it is fascinating and tempting. Seed grain is treated with mercury and, if eaten by mistake, can cause severe symptoms. There are many other sources of mercury, including some cosmetics, latex and solvent-thinned paints, fabric softeners, floor polishes, air-conditioning filters and fungicides used in the garden. Fatigue, memory loss and headaches are common symptoms. The more severe symptoms can mimic those of multiple sclerosis, including numbness and tingling, poor coordination, impaired sight and hearing, emotional disturbances, difficulty with speech and eventually kidney damage, seriously impaired brain function and death.

Vitamin C helps to protect you from the damage of these elements, but like all the toxic metals, the best solution is avoidance.

These are just a few of the toxic metals in the environment. As you can see, many of them induce fatigue and lethargy. All of them have symptoms that can seriously overload the body's ability to eliminate the toxins; all of them can do serious damage and act as a significant drain on your resources. Do all you can to avoid these toxins. If you think you have been exposed to one or more of them, the Hair Tissue Mineral test is a good idea (see Chapter Seven). When you get the result, you will be given a list of possible sources and a suggested treatment programme.

Social Drugs

How often have you finished a day's work, sat down to unwind and had a drink – something alcoholic to help you relax and give you the get-up-and-go to start preparing dinner or to revive you for the evening ahead? Alcohol may seem to relax you and give you energy, yet can actually increase your fatigue. Alcohol interferes with a number of nutrients. It greatly increases your need for all the B vitamins, as your liver works at detoxifying or metabolising the alcohol, and we have already seen how important they are for energy production. Alcohol can interfere with absorption of nutrients. Low-alcohol drinks, such as wine and beer that contain yeast, encourage candida and we will soon see what a devastating effect this can have on your energy level (Chapter Sixteen). One heavy evening's drinking can wipe out all the vitamin B12 you have stored in your liver, which might otherwise have amounted to several days', or even a week or two's supply. Thus anaemia is a possible consequence of a heavy drinking bout.

Cigarettes severely deplete the body of a variety of nutrients necessary for the production of energy. Smokers need extra vitamin A, zinc and lecithin for the lining of the lungs and most of the B vitamins to support the liver in dealing with the various chemicals that are both present and produced in and by the inhaled smoke. Each cigarette increases your need for vitamin C, possibly by 100 mg or more per cigarette.

Medical Drugs

Overall, there are many drugs that interfere with energy levels; in fact, very few don't. Many of them interfere with vitamin metabolism[1] and thus have an adverse effect on your health and energy. Others interfere with

DNA metabolism and thus can contribute to megaloblastic anaemia and hence energy loss.

Neomycin, an antibiotic, can reduce vitamin B12 absorption.

The contraceptive pill reduces vitamin absorption, including absorption of B9 and so can lead to anaemia. It also increases your need for vitamin B6.

Diuretics are used to increase the loss of fluids from the body. Unfortunately, they also increase the loss of a variety of water-soluble substances including essential nutrients such as vitamins and minerals. It is common to find that you have been given a potassium supplement in combination with the diuretic since doctors recognise this connection. However, they rarely suggest supplementing with any of the other nutrients your body loses as a direct result of the diuretic. Further, the form of potassium given, potassium chloride, can interfere with vitamin B12 absorption and increase the risk of anaemia.

There are very few medical drugs that do not greatly increase your need for nutrients and entire books have been written on the subject.

What To Do

Everybody is exposed to environmental toxins and hazards. It is simply a question of degree. You should therefore protect yourself as much as you can from the harm they can do to you, and you can do this in a number of ways. One of the first things you may ask is 'which are the worst toxins?' A more useful question is 'which toxins can I most easily avoid?' Even if you remove minor ones, if you remove enough of them you will be reducing the total toxic load significantly and this is important. Avoid all the toxins you possibly can. From the above, you may already have identified a number of factors in your environment that could be causing problems.

I have one colleague who had to build himself a small cabin in the garden of their weekend house in the country. After a year of living there in isolation, all his many health problems disappeared and, provided he maintained his supplement programme and avoided the worst pollutants, he was eventually able to rejoin the family. This is obviously a severe case. However, if you are suffering from CFS and have not be able to get your energy back, no matter what you have tried, it may be necessary – and it is certainly better than years of exhaustion. The problem may not be this severe for you, so take heart. If your energy loss is severe, and before you decide that it is all too much trouble, you should consider that the rewards could be a lot greater than you anticipate, both in increased energy, health, well-being and longevity, and well worth the effort.

After you have done all you can to ensure either avoidance or minimal exposure, get to work on your own body. Put it through a cleansing programme. Clean out the digestive tract and restore the normal flora and function. Full details for doing this are given in Part IV (Chapter Twenty-seven). However, there are a variety of steps you can take if the situation is not so severe.

If you feel so inclined, go on a water or fruit juice fast for a few days. There are many excellent books giving you the detailed procedures for this. Alternatively, spend a few days living on fresh fruit and vegetables and drinking fruit and vegetable juices. Ideally, of course, they should be organically grown. You should also be taking broad spectrum multivitamin and mineral supplements and, as part of a detox programme, an additional supplement of antioxidants. Your health-food store should be able to provide this. If even this programme seems too extreme for you, then at least do all you can to improve your diet. Cut out processed foods, fried foods, saturated fats and sugars. Drink at least three pints of purified water a day, either as water, fruit juice, herb teas or coffee substitutes. Cut out tea, coffee and alcohol.

Take a supplement of *lactobacillus acidophilus*. Drink 50 ml of pure aloe vera juice three times a day. If you experience heartburn, intestinal pain or discomfort, take a teaspoon of slippery elm powder night and morning. An easy way to get this down is to mash it into half a banana. The slippery elm powder forms an internal bandage and the aloe and the zinc, vitamin A and vitamin E in the supplements you take will encourage healing. If you think you might be short of stomach acids, take a supplement containing some hydrochloric acid.

If you want to check whether or not toxic minerals are a problem, you can do so by having a hair mineral analysis done. This normally checks on your levels of lead, mercury, cadmium, aluminium and arsenic at least. If you find that you have a toxic load of one or more of these minerals, do what you can to identify the source and avoid it, and take the appropriate nutrients to counterbalance the problem.

Toxins always put a heavy stress on the liver, so add eggs (yes, eggs – the cholesterol is not the problem it has been made out to be, as we shall see in Chapter Nineteen) to your diet, since they are rich in the protective, sulphur-rich amino acids, methionine and cysteine; take all the B group vitamins; and add lecithin to your diet. You may be able to buy a supplement specifically designed to protect and support the liver.

Give up alcohol. When you drink alcohol, your detox mechanisms deal with the alcohol before they deal with a variety of other toxins which can accumulate and do their damage. Alcohol also puts a stress on the liver, a very important organ for dealing with toxins, and uses up valuable nutrients, badly needed by the rest of your detox mechanisms.

The majority of toxic chemicals are either oxidising agents or they generate free radicals. Free radicals are highly reactive bits of molecules. They are not complete molecules, nor are they the normally-charged ions that are components of molecules. Instead, it is as if a molecule has been wrenched in two and is doing all it can to get back together again. In the process, it will collide with and damage thousands of other molecules. The net result is significant damage not only to the molecules with which it reacts directly, but to the surrounding tissues. Many of these free radicals are also oxidising agents. For this reason, it is important that you take a lot of antioxidants, particularly vitamins A, C and E, beta carotine and the bioflavonoids, and the minerals selenium, copper (if you need it, see Chapter Seven) manganese and zinc, and eat foods rich in these nutrients.

No matter what your state of health, you will benefit from eliminating toxins from your lifestyle as far as you possibly can. If you are feeling tired and run down, a detox programme will provide additional benefit.

For further information, see *A Clinician's guide to Toxic Metals, sources, occupation exposures, signs and symptoms.* MineralLab Inc, 3501 Breakwater Avenue, Hayward, California.

---

[1] See Roe, D., *Drug-induced nutritional deficiencies.* Avi Publishing Company, 1978.

Chapter Nine

———————————————————

Anaemia

General

Most people are aware that iron deficiency can cause anaemia and that when you are anaemic you will almost certainly feel tired. Fewer people are aware that anaemia does not *necessarily* mean you have an iron deficiency. Anaemia can also be caused by a deficiency of copper, folic acid, vitamin B6, vitamin B12, vitamin C, vitamin E and a number of other nutrients. It also has causes that are not necessarily related directly to the diet or your nutritional status. A deficiency of iron, folic acid and vitamin B12 are thought to be the main causes of anaemia, but if you are suffering from anaemia and it does not respond to treatment or supplementation with these nutrients then consider the other nutrients listed above. Of course, they should be part of your general supplementation programme.

In addition to anaemia, an iron deficiency can cause tiredness in many other ways, as we have seen (Chapter Seven). In this chapter, however, we shall focus on anaemia.

IRON AND ANAEMIA
Energy Production

Since we are discussing iron and anaemia in regard to the energy you have, it is appropriate to take an overview of the way energy is produced in the body as it relates to your iron levels.

Ultimately, the energy you have comes from the breakdown of the foods you eat. Your food, whether it is of good or poor quality, in the right or the wrong proportions, consists of fats, proteins and carbohydrates, which are broken down in the digestive tract, absorbed, transported through the bloodstream and, eventually, delivered to the cells as fatty acids, glucose and amino acids, all of which are then available for energy generation via combustion.

Through various series of reactions, or metabolic pathways, and with the assistance of a number of vitamins and trace elements as cofactors, these substances, once inside the cells, are broken down further and their energy is released. This part of the process involves the oxygen in the air that you breathe. This oxygen is carried to the cells where it combines with the carbon atoms in the foods to form carbon dioxide as the final waste product. This is then transported through the blood to the lungs and you expel it when you breathe out. The oxygen from the air also combines with the hydrogen atoms in the foods to form water as the final waste product. This is transported via the blood to the kidneys, where it is passed out as urine. The nitrogen in the amino acids does not provide energy so it need not concern us here. It is simply 'made safe' via the liver and kidneys and it too is secreted in the urine. For our purposes, it is important that by the action of the oxygen in the air you breathe in, food is converted into carbon dioxide, water and energy.

For these reactions to occur, the oxygen obviously has to be carried from the lungs, through the bloodstream and delivered into the cells where these final reactions take place. This oxygen then has to be available within the cell's powerhouses, the mitochondria, in the amount required to generate energy. Overall there are two parts to this process. One part involves the transport of oxygen from the walls of the lungs through the bloodstream and into the cells that need the energy. The other part involves the action of that oxygen on the fatty acids, glucose and amino acids within the cells. Many nutrients, including iron, are involved in both these sequences of reactions.

Anaemia

Anaemia is defined as 'a deficiency in the blood, either in quality or quantity'. It usually refers to a deficiency in the number of red blood cells or to low levels of haemoglobin, the red blood pigment that contains iron and carries the oxygen. Anaemia is generally regarded not so much as a disease in itself as a symptom of a variety of different disorders.

The many different types of anaemia can all lead to fatigue and lassitude. They can exist and contribute to your symptoms long before the normal medical blood tests show your results to be outside the normal range. The process is a gradual one as your red cell activity moves slowly away from the point that is normal for you, whether or not it is within the average spectrum for most people. Blood tests will only detect a condition when it is sufficiently severe to show up as a significant pathology. Long before this happens, you may begin to feel tired and run down, gradually feeling worse and worse until tests eventually confirm the condition. Our challenge is to identify the problem before it becomes this severe and to set it in its wider context.

Anaemia through Loss of Blood

Loss of blood as a cause of anaemia is so obvious you might think it would be hard to miss, yet this can happen. The loss can be due to menstruation, to 'invisible' loss from the digestive tract, to internal bleeding or to overt loss through the skin. Some of this bleeding, such as menstrual bleeding, is so normal, it is easy to take it for granted and overlook the fact that you may not be replacing the blood as fast as you lose it.

Robin came into the office saying she was exhausted, and yet there seemed to be no obvious cause. What could be the problem? She did add that she was getting a few hot flushes: could it be that the menopause was starting? Only after some time had elapsed did she mention that she was having another problem, painful and difficult periods. On further discussion she agreed that her periods had also been unusually heavy of late, but added that they were always pretty heavy and so she had thought little of it. After thirty years of relatively heavy monthly bleeds with possible insufficient replacement of the blood lost, and increasingly heavy flows as she went into the menopause, she could indeed have been short of blood, short of iron and on the verge of anaemia. The fact that the flow during last few months had been unusually heavy may have been the last straw.

Young adolescent girls who are growing and menstruating may become anaemic because of menstrual blood loss combined with an increased demand for blood as they grow. Pregnant women and women who bleed each month obviously need to absorb more iron than women who don't menstruate, or men. New blood can be made in the body, but not iron. It has to be absorbed from food, hence the need for additional amounts in the diet.

Martin Roberts had a different problem. He had had a stomach ulcer for three years, but claimed it was under control with medication. The current problem was his tiredness and inability to keep up with the workload the way he used to in his very stressful financial job. After detailed questioning it emerged that he frequently had stools that were very dark, sometimes nearly black. On testing this turned out to be due to a high content of blood. It is likely that his ulcers, while no longer causing pain, were still bleeding, and it is possible for a significant amount of blood loss to occur in this way. His fatigue was a natural consequence of this.

If blood loss is severe, transfusion may be needed. If there has been no major trauma, it is more likely that you need first to stop the loss of blood and then to focus on the nutrients needed to ensure the healthy production of new blood. If your periods are heavy, on a regular basis, then ensure that you take a supplement with iron, folic acid and vitamin B12. There are other natural treatments for the problem itself, but that is another story.

Iron Deficiency Anaemia

Iron deficiency is a major cause of anaemia and probably the best known. A lack of iron may be something you associate with underdeveloped societies but it is relatively common in the western world. Your doctor may tell you it is the most common mineral deficiency found, but it is often the only mineral they look for so this is not truly significant.

A deficiency may be caused by lack of iron in the

diet, by poor absorption of iron, possibly associated with inadequate acid production in the stomach, by poor absorption across the intestinal walls, by inadequate transport through the blood, or inadequate uptake of iron into the red cells (see Chapter Seven). To decide how you are going to correct these problems you should refer back to Chapters Three and Seven.

Darkfield Test

There is a useful test, carried out by an increasing number of natural therapists, known as the Darkfield Test. Individual live cells are looked at against a dark background, to obtain information relating to the adequacy of your stomach acid levels, the fluidity of your blood, your overall nutrient status, whether or not your cells are being affected by oxidising agents (in which case you need more antioxidants), the health of your liver, the tendency of your red blood cells to stick together or clot and more, much more.

From our point of view, the test is useful as it can tell you much about the possibility of anaemia and, should it exist, the type of anaemia you may have. If the red cells are small, it is microcytic anaemia and you could need iron; if they are large, it is macrocytic and you could need vitamin B12, as we shall see; if the white blood cells commonly have four or more nuclei, you could also benefit from folic acid and vitamin B12. If the red cells have light rings in them, you are probably iron deficient. However if you cannot have this test done, remember the signs of iron deficiency, and hence anaemia, given in Chapter Seven.

Microcytic Anaemia

This type of anaemia can be caused by reduced production of haemoglobin, the central compound in the red cells and the compound that includes iron, and then combines with oxygen as this enters the blood from the lungs. In this type of anaemia the blood will be paler than usual and the red cells smaller. You can look for the external signs that were described in Chapter Seven.

Since iron deficiency is the most common cause, we will consider how it can arise. Clearly the amount of iron in the diet has to be adequate; without that nothing else will improve the situation. Iron requirements increase during pregnancy, although even here the amount present may be adequate but its absorption and usage may be compromised. Requirements are also increased if there has been increased blood loss – either external as a result of accident or trauma, or internal such as from ulcers or colitis or during increased menstrual bleeding.

Commonly, however, in a diet with a significant amount of meat and other iron rich foods, it is not the intake of iron that is the problem but its absorption and utilisation. Malabsorption can come about if there are problems in the digestive tract, such as if part of the digestive tract is missing – for example, after an operation. Parasites such as worms can also reduce iron absorption. Poor absorption, transport and usage of iron can come about as a result of a lack of other important nutrients required for these purposes and for the production of haemoglobin, including several B group vitamins and vitamin C.

Certain drugs such as some used against tuberculosis and cancer, chemicals such as alcohol, and other toxins such as lead are also known to cause microcytic anaemia. Further, there are many other, relatively exotic, diseases associated with microcytic anaemia but if you had these it is likely, though not certain, that your health care practitioner would already have picked them up.

Obviously iron is needed, but it is also important to provide the B group vitamins involved in the usage of iron and its incorporation into the red blood cells. This means taking vitamin B6, B12 and folic acid. Vitamin C helps in the absorption of iron and, if digestion is poor, a hydrochloric acid supplement may be needed. The iron and B-vitamin content of the diet should also be increased by including meat and dark green, leafy vegetables. It is worth noting that the iron from meat is absorbed very much more effectively than the iron from vegetables, possibly as much as ten or fifteen times as effectively.

Macrocytic Anaemia

This is, in some ways, the opposite of microcytic in that this time the red blood cells are larger than normal. This type of anaemia is more common when there is a deficiency of folic acid or vitamin B12. This results in deficient amounts of RNA and DNA, the genetic material within cells, and the red cells increase in size before their growth stops and new cell growth starts. These large red cells are less robust than the standard ones and die more rapidly. As a result, they are less able to transport adequate amounts of oxygen to your cells.

There are many factors behind this type of anaemia. It can be caused by excess alcohol intake and by problems in the liver such as obstructive jaundice, cirrhosis or hepatitis. Hormonal causes include hypothyroidism. It can occur after the spleen is removed, when there is increased hemolysis (breakdown) of the red cells, during bleeding, and is associated with some other, less common diseases.

A lack of vitamin B12 in the diet can cause this type of anaemia and so can poor B12 absorption which has already been discussed (Chapter Six). As always with absorption it is important to ensure that there is no damage to the intestinal wall. If there is a folic acid or B12 deficiency then damage is likely as these vitamins are needed for DNA and RNA activity and so for regenerating new cells. This means you can get an escalating problem: a lack of folic acid and B12 leading to damaged cells, including those lining the stomach (and so to a lack of intrinsic factor synthesis: see Chapter Six) and small intestine which then leads to decreased absorption, which further worsens the situation.

A number of drugs can inhibit B12 absorption, both medical drugs and alcohol, which should be avoided. Ironically the potassium chloride given to people on diuretics also inhibits B12 absorption.

People needing B12 are normally given an injection once a month, since it can be stored in the liver for many weeks. This has sometimes lead people to assume that, since the liver can carry a large store, a deficiency is unlikely. However, this store can be lost – for instance, after only one night's heavy drinking of alcohol.

A lack of folic acid can come from a lack in the diet. It occurs in green leafy vegetables and few people eat enough of those. Its absorption can be hindered by problems in the digestive tract, including many of the more common problems in the intestines plus less common disorders such as coeliac disease and gluten sensitivity. Alcohol, the oral contraceptive pill, anti-convulsants and a number of other drugs and chemicals decrease absorption of folic acid, as do cirrhosis of the liver and a variety of enzyme deficiencies.

It is important to ensure that you provide *all* the nutrients that are needed. If you suspect you are lacking in vitamin B12, this may well be true, but you may have other deficiencies as well. I recall the case of one woman who thought a vitamin B12 shot had solved all her problems and then found out that it hadn't.

Margaret had been feeling tired for a couple of years, since a miscarriage, and had eventually been given a B12 shot by her doctor. The effect, she said, had been marvellous. Within days she had felt wonderful, full of energy and back to the way she had felt years before the miscarriage. Then her energy had fallen again, she'd gone back to the doctor for another shot and felt fantastic. She found that a monthly shot had kept her energy up for nearly a year. Then they seemed to stop working and the doctor said there was nothing more he could do.

Together, we worked out a diet that would give her better nutrition and combined that with a total supplement programme. Once more, she improved and felt wonderful for months; then, as before, her energy deserted her. She then worked at improving her absorption and took hydrochloric acid and enzymes. Again, her energy improved, but only for a few months. When I suggested that she might need the B12 shots as well as the general supplement and enzymes, she was at first reluctant to consider it, insisting she had tried that and it hadn't worked, she had tried multivitamins and they hadn't worked, and she was losing faith. However, she agreed to try again. This time the combination of B12 shots (and remember that for some people it can be difficult to absorb this vitamin orally), enzymes and a general nutritional supplement did the trick. Now, two years later, this combination has continued to provide her with all the energy she needs to run her home and family plus a full-time career. She needs a B12 shot only about twice a year, but she does need to keep them going at that level.

Each time her body ran out of a nutrient, Margaret felt tired. When the weakest link in the chain was fixed she was fine until her reserves were exhausted and the next-weakest link showed up. While a single nutrient deficiency may often be the immediate cause of your fatigue, the answer is often, as in Margaret's case, more complex. So if your first attempts aren't totally success-ful, keep trying.

Other Nutrients

Iron, folic acid and vitamin B12 are not the only nutrients needed to ensure the absence of anaemia and the proper delivery of oxygen to the cells. As already mentioned, you should ensure your diet is adequate in all respects.

Exercise

It has been found that the iron status of long distance runners is usually poor. This can mean that, in spite of all their training, they can be iron-deficient with or without anaemia, and have less energy than they want or need. In other words, a group of people that you would expect to be fit and energetic can have less than the expected amount of energy simply because of the physical activity they do. The iron status of female runners is particularly likely to be compromised because of menstruation, and in fact menstruation often ceases in these athletes. Treat-ment with iron is often unsuccessful as their transferin saturation level (part of the mechanism in the small intestine walls alluded to in Chapter Seven) is often high.

Exercise can cause breakdown of the red blood cells simply because they have to process such large amounts of oxygen to generate the energy required. This in turn can lead to an increase in free radical activity. The answer may be both to give iron supplements and to supplement with coenzyme Q10 as a free radical scavenger, plus other antioxidants such as carotene, vitamins A, C and E and the minerals copper, manganese, selenium and zinc.

When a person suffers a heart attack, there is damage to the muscles of the heart. This results in an increased release of certain enzymes into the bloodstream, specifically to increased levels of an enzyme called CPK. The level of this enzyme in the blood is used as one of the measures of a heart attack, its timing and its severity. This same enzyme is released from other muscles when they break down and athletes who put severe strain on their muscles may often show blood levels of this enzyme as high as those of heart attack patients. To prevent this muscle breakdown, damage and exhaustion you need those antioxidants again, and especially vitamin E.

Symptoms

Obviously anaemia can lead to tiredness, lethargy and apathy. It is very hard to keep going when your cells are not generating energy. If you are tired, it may be because you are anaemic. Other symptoms include general pallor, pale inside lower eye-lids, pale nail beds and pale palmar creases when extended (see Chapter Seven for other signs of iron deficiency).

What To Do

Check for the signs given above that might suggest you are anaemic.

- Take an organic iron supplement, not ferrous sulphate (see Chapter Seven).
- Make sure the supplement includes folic acid and vitamin B12.

- Take a supplement of hydrochloric acid (in tablet form) at least for a month.
- Take a month's supply of stomach and pancreatic digestive enzymes as separate supplements.
- Take a course of acidophilus and bifidus to help to improve the intestinal flora so that more vitamin B12 is synthesised and less is consumed by organisms.

Unless there are overt signs (Chapter Three) of the need for stomach acid, digestive enzymes and acidophilus, these can be stopped once the signs of anaemia have gone. You may need to continue the iron, folic acid and vitamin B12 supplement – though possibly at a lower dose – to prevent the return of the problem. You should also increase the iron content of your diet (see Chapter Seven).

Chapter Ten

The Thyroid Gland

One of the hormone systems that is essential for the normal production and maintenance of energy is the system associated with the thyroid gland.

Perhaps you have met people who are lethargic, never having enough energy no matter what they eat or do, who are overweight, swearing they only have to think of food to gain weight (and we will assume here that they are being honest and not cheating and *still* gaining weight), and who feel the cold and wear an extra layer of clothing.

You may also know some people who are always on the go, seeming to have an excess of nervous energy, always doing things and rarely sitting still. They can eat anything they want and stay as thin as a rake and they are always throwing the blankets off the bed, feeling hot and frequently sweating.

The first group may be suffering from an underactive thyroid gland and the second from an overactive thyroid. It is no fun being tired and lethargic. Equally, it is no fun having so much energy you don't know what to do with it and feeling like a coiled spring with nowhere to go.

The Hypothalamic–Pituitary–Thyroid Connection

The story starts in the hypothalamus, a tiny gland weighing about seven grams or a quarter of an ounce, hidden in a cavity within the brain. For all its small size, it wields extraordinary power, in many ways controlling the activity of all the other glands, including the thyroid.

The hypothalamus also functions as a major link between the mind and the body. It allows for thoughts and emotions to be translated into changes within the body, for anxieties to result in that sinking feeling in your stomach, for nervousness and fear to result in shaking hands, for shock at some news to lower your skin temperature and for anger to trigger off reactions in the stomach that can lead to ulcers. It is via the hypothalamus that your fears and anxieties can actually turn into psychosomatic illnesses and your positive thoughts and determination to win can help you beat a seemingly insurmountable health problem.

It is the hypothalamus that sends out instructions affecting the thyroid gland. The hypothalamus takes in all the messages it receives (we will consider these later) and when it thinks the thyroid should be working harder, it sends out a compound called Thyroid-Releasing-Hormone (TRH), made up of several amino acids joined in a peptide chain. This hormone goes to the pituitary gland and passes on its message that greater thyroid activity is required.

The pituitary gland is also situated within the brain and is also a very tiny gland – even smaller in fact, than the hypothalamus, weighing in at only half a gram or one-sixtieth of an ounce. Yet it controls so many body functions that you'd be totally lost without it. When the pituitary receives Thyroid-Releasing Hormone (TRH) from the hypothalamus, it in turn secretes a compound called Thyroid-Stimulating-Hormone (TSH), another molecule made of amino acids, and sends this, in turn, to the thyroid gland.

Your thyroid gland is situated in the front of your neck just below your larynx or voice-box and is made up of two wings or lobes, one on either side of the trachea or windpipe. It has two jobs to do. One is to release calcitonin when it is needed. Calcitonin is involved with calcium metabolism and so does not concern us here. The other job the thyroid does is to release the correct amount of thyroxin hormones into the bloodstream. These then go to the cells througout the body and instruct them to burn up more fuel, create more energy and be more active. There are two of these hormones, technically called tri-iodo-thyronine (T3) and tetra-iodo-thyronine (T4). T4 is the main one and is often called, simply, 'thyroxin'.

Both T3 and the more common T4 have an amino acid base, with either three or four atoms of iodine attached, (see Chapter Seven), and when you are tired and rundown and an underactive thyroid is suspected, you will often be advised to take either a supplement of iodine or, more usually, some kelp, which is a rich source of iodine.

When the appropriate triggers are received and thyroxin is released, it goes to the various cells throughout the body and stimulates them to take in more oxygen from the haemoglobin passing by in the red blood cells. With this extra oxygen, the cells are able to burn up the stored fats and carbohydrates and generate energy. It is rather like using a bellows to blow more air (oxygen) into the fire to stimulate the burning of the wood and thus the generation of heat (energy).

When the energy production reaches the desired level, the hypothalamus can relax. When insufficient energy is being produced and there is insufficient thyroxin circulating in the blood, the hypothalamus will get the message and become active; it will send out more Thyroid-Releasing Hormone (TRH) and the cycle starts over again.

Too Much Thyroxin

When there is too much thyroxin, the cells start burning up both your stores of spare fat and the protein of your muscles. In the analogy with a fire, this would be like the fire burning up not only the wood pile but also the furniture and structures of the house – obviously not a desirable situation. To avoid this loss of body tissue, the person with an overactive thyroid gland usually has a big appetite. Since the food is being consumed in this raging furnace in the cells, the person will not gain weight. They will, however, have more energy than they know what to do with and feel uncomfortable. They will also sweat a lot and be hot to touch. If they fail to eat they will continue to burn up needed stores of fat and muscle and will lose weight. If this continues they will also lose strength as their muscles become weak.

In the brain an excess of thyroxin causes increased mental activity, irritability and tension. Thoughts will be flying round in your head and you will feel restless.

Thyroxin stimulates the formation of cholesterol within your body. It also increases the removal of cholesterol from your body via the liver and the large bowel. Since this removal outweighs production, the net effect of excessive production of thyroxin is to lower your blood cholesterol levels. This has a useful corollary. A high cholesterol level should alert you to the possibility of an underactive thyroid and encourage you to try the test described later in this chapter.

Too Little Thyroxin

When there is too little thyroxin in your blood the cells
do not draw in sufficient oxygen from the haemoglobin
passing by in the red blood cells. Without this oxygen,
just like fire without air, the cells cannot burn up their
fuel (in this case the carbohydrates and fats) and do not
generate energy and so become sluggish. As a result you
too become tired and sluggish.

Many people eat when they feel tired, feeling that this
will give them a lift. It often doesn't, because nothing has
been done to stimulate the cells to increased metabolic
activity. If your thyroid is underactive, your cells are not
sluggish for lack of fuel – they have plenty of that. It is
the oxygen release, the action of thyroxin, that is missing.
All your body can do with this extra food you eat is to
convert it into fat stores and deposit it in all those places
where you normally store fats, such as the thighs and
buttocks, in the hope that at some time in the future
there will be sufficient thyroxin activity for the cells to
use it for the production of energy. As a result, of course,
you get fat – and remain tired.

Other things happen too when your thyroid gland
is underactive. Your skin contains carbohydrate–protein
complexes. If your thyroid is underactive these accumulate and promote water retention. As a result your skin
becomes bloated and puffy. Because the cells are not
generating energy and heat, you feel cold, and your
body feels cold to the touch.

One set of cells that is less active under these conditions is your bone marrow, where the blood cells are
produced. Another set is the cells in the stomach lining
that produce the Intrinsic Factor, the substance that helps
you to absorb vitamin B 12. The result is anaemia and
this too makes you feel tired, as we have already seen.

The liver cells become less active and as a result they

fail to convert beta-carotene, the orange colour in carrots and similar foods, into vitamin A so you can become vitamin A deficient. Further, the carotenes, being yellow (whereas vitamin A is not), are left intact and give the skin a yellowish colour. This is different from jaundice. In jaundice the skin is also yellow but the whites of the eyes turn yellow too; this does not happen with an accumulation of beta-carotene.

Normal thyroxin production is essential for adequate production of breast milk. If you are lactating and tired your milk flow may be reduced. You may put this down to being tired, and in a sense you would be correct, but in fact both could be a consequence of insufficient thyroxin production. Thyroxin plays a role in the normal menstrual cycle and in fertility. You may have problems in that area and put them down to the stresses in your life and being tired, but again, both the tiredness and the menstrual problems or infertility may actually stem from low thyroxin levels.

In the brain low levels of thyroxin lead to mental sluggishness, the opposite of the effect of high levels. You may think more slowly, have less initiative and feel less like doing things than when your thyroid levels are normal.

Another problem with low thyroxin levels relates to your sex drive which is likely to fall as the thyroxin levels do. You may think your interest in sex has waned simply because you are tired. In fact, both your sex drive and your energy may independently be low because of an underactive thyroid gland.

How To Know

If you are wondering about your own thyroid gland and whether or not it is functioning at the correct rate, there are a couple of things you can do. You can of course go to your doctor and ask to have a blood test done to find out. This will show the levels of T3, T4 and TSH and provide other relevant information. The problem is that quite a wide range of results is considered to be 'normal', since people vary as to what is an optimal level for them.

The problem occurs if your own normal level is close to the upper edge of the normal range and your result comes in at the lower edge. The doctor will tell you that the results are within the normal range. What he won't tell you, and cannot know, is that for you this is significantly below normal. In effect, this test may only pick up the problem when it has become severe. There is a further problem with the quoted normal levels for these tests as we will see shortly, but first let's consider a simple test you can do at home with a simple thermometer.

This test has been well researched and described by an American doctor, Dr Broda Barnes with Lawrence Galton in *Hypothyroidism: The unsuspected illness* (Thos. Y. Crowell Co., 666 Fifth Avenue, New York City, 10019). The test involves measuring your temperature when you are as close as possible to your resting, basal metabolic rate. The way to do this is to take your temperature under your armpit when you are as relaxed as you possibly can be. If you sleep on your own, then shake the thermometer down the night before, so it is ready to use. When you first become slightly conscious in the morning, put the thermometer under your arm and try to relax back into a doze; sleep if you can. After about ten minutes, take the thermometer out and write down the reading exactly. If you are male you can do this on any two or three days in the month. If you are female you should, ideally, do it on the second and third days of menstruation because basal temperature changes during the menstrual cycle. If you are impatient, do it anyway, but reserve your final judgement until you've measured it on these two days.

Normal basal temperature is within the range of 97.8 to 98.2°F or 36.55 to 36.78°C. So if your temperature is below either 97.8°F or 36.55°C, you probably have an underactive thyroid. The degree of underactivity may not be sufficient to produce serious clinical symptoms and negative signs on a blood test, but it could well be sufficient to be the cause of your tiredness and lack of energy.

Dr Barnes believes that around forty per cent of the population has an underactive thyroid. If this is the case and if you feel tired, there is a relatively high chance that your thyroid is not doing its job properly. This also highlights another inadequacy of the blood tests for thyroid function. If such a high proportion of the population is hypothyroid, then many people whose levels are actually low were probably considered to be 'normal' and their results incorporated into the information used to establish the 'normal' levels used and quoted by doctors. It may well be that the levels set as 'normal' for the blood tests are in fact too low and fail to show up a significant number of people who would benefit from moves to increase their thyroid activity.

You should also check out the symptoms that are associated with low thyroid activity. In descending order of frequency, these are weakness, dry skin, coarse skin, lethargy, slow speech, oedema of the eyelids, feeling cold, reduced sweating, cold skin, thick tongue, facial oedema, coarseness of hair, enlarged heart, pale skin, poor memory, constipation, weight gain, loss of hair, pale lips, laboured or difficult breathing, swelling of the feet and hoarseness, plus (according to a second study) slow movements, muscle weakness, depression and burning or tingling sensations (J.H. Means, L.J. DeGroot and J.B. Sainsbury, *The Thyroid and its Diseases*, McGraw-Hill, 1963, pp. 321–22).

What To Do

If you have a number of the symptoms of an underactive thyroid and your basal temperature is low, you will want to know what has to be done to raise the activity of this gland and so increase your energy. The first thing you might do is have a blood test and determine the level of the thyroid factors. This will give you a yardstick for possible use and comparison in the future. Remember, however, that even if they are within the range quoted as normal, for you this is too low. The evidence is that you should believe and work with your basal temperature and your symptoms rather than with these blood test results.

Important supplements include iodine, since it is an essential part of the thyroxin molecule. One of the best ways to take it is in the form of kelp. Other nutrients are also important. Copper is needed by the thyroid gland. If your water pipes are made of copper, you probably have sufficient, but if your water pipes are made of galvanised iron, plastic or some other material then you could need a copper supplement.

Manganese is another important trace mineral. This is seriously lacking in Australian soils, less so in those of Great Britain and Europe. As already mentioned (Chapter Seven), in two studies of over one hundred people each, in Australia, I found that manganese deficiency was extremely common. Part of the problem may be that people often take a zinc supplement without combining it with manganese, thus creating a manganese deficiency as there is competition between the two minerals. It is thought that the ratio of zinc to manganese intake, in normal health, should be around fourteen to one – although this depends on your starting levels of each nutrient and your own particular metabolism. If you are lacking in manganese but have sufficient zinc, you will need to increase the relative intake of manganese. One way to determine a possible manganese deficiency is by Hair Mineral Analysis.

Low levels of vitamin A can interfere with the normal function of T3 and T4. This vitamin is found in foods of animal origin such as meat and liver. Plant foods generally thought of as being rich in vitamin A – foods such as carrots, pumpkins, apricots and dark green vegetables – are actually rich in beta-carotene. Beta-carotene is two molecules of vitamin A joined together and so should, at least in theory, deliver vitamin A to the body when it is broken down. Unfortunately, not everyone is efficient in dividing the beta-carotene in half. This means that some vegetarians could be vitamin A-deficient even though they do eat a lot of carotene. This is a point worth considering if you are a tired vegetarian.

A lack of vitamin E reduces iodine absorption. So it could be that you have taken kelp and still didn't feel more energetic. Then, for some reason, you might take a vitamin E supplement. You could then conclude that you didn't need the kelp, only the vitamin E, but that would be wrong. You could well have needed both.

In addition to food you should eat and supplements you should take, there are some foods you should avoid if your thyroid activity is low. These include those in the brassica family such as cabbage, brussel sprouts, cauliflower and broccoli, which tend to slow thyroid activity, and soy beans and peanuts which can reduce iodine absorption.

There are homeopathic remedies that stimulate the thyroid back to normal function. These can be obtained from a homeopath or suppliers of homeopathic remedies. It is also possible, in some countries, such as America, to get tablets made from desiccated thyroid.

You could also take thyroxin, the pure hormone, either extracted from an animal source or made synthetically, and prescribed by your doctor, but that is not something I recommend. Firstly, you will have to find a doctor who understands the importance and relevance of your resting temperature and understands that even if your blood levels of thyroid hormones and related factors are within the range that is considered to be normal, you may in fact be hypothyroid.

The secondary problems and considerations are even more important. When you take a tablet containing the thyroxin hormone, this hormone moves through the bloodstream in a similar way to your own thyroxin. It also passes through the brain, giving the message to the hypothalamus that enough of it is present. The hypothalamus has no way of detecting that the thyroxin has come from an outside source. It 'assumes' that its own actions have generated it; it may even think it has triggered the synthesis of an excessive amount and therefore slow down its own action in releasing TRH. This will, in turn, slow down the pituitary's production of TSH and this will curtail your own synthesis and release of thyroxin. All this will lead to a negative spiral and a greater dependence on external thyroxin.

Patients often ask if taking vitamin and mineral supplements can have a similar negative feed-back effect. It cannot since you do not manufacture them at all in the first place and thus have no feedback mechanism telling you whether or not you have made sufficient. If you are deficient in vitamins and minerals, take them. Your body will use them and you will benefit.

The problem with taking thyroxin from some external, animal source is that you are not solving the real problem, your own inadequate production of thyroxin. But by using the other methods described above you are helping to solve the basic, causative problem.

If all else fails, if your thyroid is still underactive and you feel you must take some physical thyroid supplement, then I would suggest the desiccated thyroid gland rather than pure thyroxin. As you read the result below from Dr Hoffer's work on cancer patients, you will understand why.

On the efficacy of natural methods and the homeopathics I can speak from personal experience. For a few years around 1970 my thyroid was seriously underactive. It was thought at the time that this resulted from an accident that occurred when I was working with radioactive compounds and someone had spilt radioactive iodine, which went unnoticed for several hours. Either the radioactive iodine itself, or the massive doses of non-radioactive iodine we were given as part of the subsequent 'treatment', was thought to have led to the problem. After a couple of years on thyroxin therapy, on which I was totally dependent, I learned of and took the appropriate homeopathic remedy combined with kelp and other nutrients and was soon off all medication, both from the doctor and, eventually, from the homeopathic supplier; a result that the doctor had told me would be impossible to achieve.

Other Aspects

As far back as 1948 Dr Loeser, a London gynaecologist reported[1] that women who were hyperthyroid (overactive thyroid) rarely got cancer (0.5%), whereas woman with an underactive thyroid, or who had had part of their thyroid removed, had a much higher incidence of cancer (4%). He also recognised that women with low thyroid activity commonly had high cholesterol levels. He worked with eighteen women who had had a radical mastectomy and gave them sufficient desiccated thyroid gland (1 to 5 tablets) to normalise the cholesterol levels and to maintain them. In other words, he was using their cholesterol level as an indication as to whether or not they were getting sufficient thyroid extract. After four years of boosting their thyroid activity there was only one recurrence of the cancer in these women, a much better than average result.

Dr Abram Hoffer in Canada has also studied the relationship of hypothyroidism to the incidence of cancer and came up with some further evidence for the use of thyroid extract. He found that while desiccated thyroid gland is effective in reducing the chance of a recurrence of cancer, the purified thyroxin hormone is not.

What does this mean? It means that if your thyroid gland is underfunctioning, not only may you be tired but you may be at risk of high cholesterol levels, possible associated heart problems, and cancer, particularly of the breast and genitals. If you correct the problem by stimulating the normal functioning of your own thyroid gland and, if necessary, taking thyroid extract, not only will you get your energy back but your overall health will improve enormously.

I have had dozens, if not hundreds, of patients over the years who have complained of being tired, have been to their doctor, had a variety of tests done, including thyroid function tests, and been told that everything was normal. When I have shared the above information with them and they have measured their resting temperature, a large number of them have recognised a low thyroid function as part of their problem and treatment with homeopathic, kelp, iodine and a general nutrient supplement has commonly solved the problem.

I would therefore suggest that, since you are obviously interested in your energy, you measure your own basal temperature. You will then either have solved the problem or be able to rule out one possible cause. If you are reading this book with someone else in mind, suggest that they measure theirs.

---

[1] 'A New Therapy for Prevention of Post-Operative Recurrences in Genital and Breast Cancer'. *British Medical Journal*, 2:1380–1383, 1954.

Chapter Eleven

Exhausted Adrenal Glands

We have seen how important the thyroid gland is for the production of energy and how intricate is the string of commands that leads to its release. Another glandular system that is also important for energy production is the one that involves the adrenals.

These adrenal glands, of which there are two, sit on top of your two kidneys like two little caps, one on either side of your spine, approximately level with your lower back. The outer and the inner parts secrete different types of hormones. The outer part or cortex secretes cortisone and related compounds plus the sex hormones and the inner part or medulla secretes adrenalin and noradrenalin.

We shall start by outlining how the system should work. Then we shall consider the symptoms of tired adrenals and what you can do about the situation.

There are a number of triggers for the release of these hormones, both chemical and from the nervous system. As for the thyroid, some of these triggers come from the hypothalamus and the pituitary gland, and there is a feedback loop. Once any of the hormones are released, they go out into the bloodstream and travel throughout the body where they affect a number of different organs and tissues in a variety of different ways.

Adrenalin

Adrenalin is generally thought of as part of the 'fight or flight' mechanism, the mechanism that provides the appropriate resources for you to deal with an emergency either by fighting hard or fleeing fast.

To this end it channels the flow of blood away from the digestive tract (you are hardly going to be eating a gourmet meal when running from danger) and away from the colon and kidneys (you have no time to go to the toilet in an emergency). Instead, it channels the flow of blood to the limbs, so that more oxygen can be delivered to the muscles of your legs and arms so that they in turn have the energy to run or grapple, and to the lungs so they can pick up more air. This is why it is so bad to eat when you are stressed or physically active. The stress triggers off the flow of adrenalin and your digestive system effectively shuts down.

It is already obvious that one result of the action of adrenalin is to stimulate the cells into action by supplying oxygen and thus stimulating their production of energy. In addition, it stimulates the release of glucose from the liver, thus providing the cells with a ready energy source. Conversely, when, later on, your blood sugar level falls, you are likely to feel weak, tired and shaky. Adrenalin also mobilises free fatty acids and stimulates metabolic activity, thus generating even more energy.

The Corticosteroids

Other hormones from the adrenal glands are also related, directly and indirectly, to the production of energy. These include hormones such as cortisone, cortisol, corticosterone and aldorsterone. Some of these affect mineral activity, others the metabolism of fats, proteins and carbohydrates.

Whereas adrenalin is important for your 'flight or fight' mechanism, the first stage of your stress response (see Chapter Fourteen) these hormones are involved in the second stage of stress management – in the endurance phase, when you have adapted to the stress and are coping with it, at least until your reserves run out (see Chapter Fourteen). They provide the ongoing energy you need.

All in all, if your adrenal glands are not getting all the nutrients they need to perform their task, you are going to be very tired indeed and very lacking in energy, both in the short and long term.

Blood Sugar Levels

It is worth focusing, for a moment, on the effect these adrenal hormones, plus other hormones, have on blood sugar levels. We will do this more thoroughly when we discuss hypoglycaemia (Chapter Fifteen), but this is a good place to make a start.

For good health, it is desirable that your blood sugar level stays within certain limits and that the level does not, if possible, go either above the normal upper limit or below the lower limit. To achieve this there are opposing groups of hormones. On the one hand, there is insulin whose job it is to push glucose from the bloodstream into the cells whenever the blood level gets too high. On the other hand, there are the adrenal hormones plus others from other glands that are stirred into activity whenever your blood sugar level falls. These hormones break down the cells' stores of glycogen, or animal starch, and release the glucose from which it is made, into the bloodstream, thus maintaining the blood sugar level within normal limits.

If insulin does not do its job properly, your blood sugar level remains high, as in diabetes. If the adrenal hormones do not do their job, your blood sugar level falls and you suffer from hypoglycaemia. Hypoglycaemia is a problem for two reasons. Firstly, the blood flowing through your brain does not deliver glucose to that organ. Secondly, the blood flowing through the rest of your body is not able to deliver glucose to the cells either. This means that you feel both mentally and physically tired. We will go into the symptoms and how to deal with them in Chapter Fifteen. For the moment, however, we need to focus on the overall result of adrenal glands that are tired or underactive. Clearly if they are, you are. So something has to be done about it.

These glands require certain nutrients in significant amounts. They are damaged if there is a shortage of pantothenic acid or vitamin B5. A slight deficiency causes a significant decrease in the normal function and a severe deficiency causes the glands to shrink and become physically damaged. One of the raw ingredients for making the hormones of the cortex is cholesterol and without pantothenic acid this conversion is impaired. Riboflavin (vitamin B2), vitamin A and vitamin E are also needed for proper adrenal function and so is the essential fatty acid, linoleic acid, which is found in oil-rich seeds.

Vitamin C is necessary for the formation and protection of adrenalin and noradrenalin.[1] When you do not have sufficient amounts of vitamin C, you cannot make sufficient adrenalin and noradrenalin. Further, the adrenalin and noradrealin you do make is not protected from oxidation and breakdown. In the absence of vitamin C, adrenalin is oxidised to adrenochrome and noradrenalin to noradrenochrome, both of which are toxic. Adrenochrome is extremely toxic. It interferes with a number of reactions and inhibits the release of energy from the breakdown of carbohydrates. In this way it affects all the cells in the body. It has also been found to affects brain chemistry and heart function.

Cortisone production is also dependent on the presence of vitamin C. Numerous studies, involving both people and animals, have shown that you handle stress, an emotion that cause activation of the adrenal glands, much more effectively if you have a plentiful supply of the B group vitamins and vitamin C plus sufficient of all the other nutrients for the body's needs.

As long ago as 1966 Addle Davis (*Let's Get Well*, Allen and Unwin) was drawing attention to the results of studies showing that rats, even though they *can* make their own vitamin C, died when exposed to severe cold but could survive under the same conditions if given large amounts of this vitamin. Guinea pigs (who *cannot* make this vitamin) were able to survive under the same conditions provided that they were given seventy-five times their normal intake of vitamin C. Among humans, a group whose adrenal glands were so exhausted, damaged or underfunctioning that they no longer responded to the stimulus of ACTH[2] from the pituitary gland, felt enormous benefit from being given even 500 mg of vitamin C daily, which in turn stimulated their adrenal glands to greater activity. She also reported on the beneficial effect of pantothenic acid (vitamin B5) on human volunteers experimentally exposed to stress. When people feel stressed and tired they are commonly irritable and moody as well. When human volunteers were deprived of pantothenic acid they showed the same symptoms.

When you are tired you are stressed. This may seem obvious to you. You may find yourself saying, with increasing frequency, that if you didn't have so much to do, if you weren't worried, if demands weren't being made of you, then you would not need so much energy.

This is probably true. Some people, however, claim that they are not stressed, that they are simply tired and lacking in energy. But the mere fact of being tired, of not being able to generate sufficient energy for your needs, puts a stress on the body, and on your adrenal glands. In general it is recognised that an overall B complex with vitamin C will generally help to improve your mood as well as your energy. If you are tired, it is probably time you fed your adrenal glands better – and not on chocolate and cream buns either, but on B group vitamins, especially B5, and vitamin C in particular, and overall good nutrition in general.

Some people resort to kicking their adrenal glands along by giving them a slug of caffeine in the form of coffee. This is only a short-term solution; it does not resolve the fundamental issue of why your adrenals were not functioning fully in the first place and it can generate problems of its own as we shall soon see (Chapter Twelve).

Thomas had lived on his nerves ever since he left school. Twenty years later, having had a variety of jobs, all involving finance and risk, he was a successful merchant banker and entrepreneur. He lived well, his children were at the best schools, he maintained a house in the country and a flat in the city, entertained frequently and spent much of his time 'doing deals'. When he came to see me, it was because he said he felt he was losing control; what had been an excitement and a challenge, had become a source of fear and worry. He no longer thrived on the atmosphere of financial tension but felt overwhelmed and exhausted by it.

Like so many people who choose to see a naturopath rather than a doctor, he had already thought of vitamins and had been taking both a general one and a B complex, which had helped, but only slightly.

*I pointed out that it was not simply that he was
overdoing things and working at too fast a pace, although
this was certainly true, but that he lived on surges of
adrenalin through his working day. When we topped up
his supplements with 250 mg of pantothenic acid and a
thousand mg of vitamin C taken three times a day, he
was able to get back to his old enjoyment of the challenges
of his work.*

*At the same time, I suggested that he slow down a
bit. He might keep going for another few years, but the
way he was working and living was a recipe for disaster.
No matter how much you love the excitement of your
job, it is wise to have a life of balance, where there is
also time for rest and relaxation. Otherwise you move
from the alarm and recovery stages of stress to that of
exhaustion (see Chapter Fourteen).*

It's not only people who lead obviously high-stress jobs
who may benefit from nutrients designed to help the
adrenal glands. I recall a secretary who was afraid of her
boss; each time he spoke to her, her 'stomach did flip-
flops', as she put it. She benefited from a B complex
with extra pantothenic acid and vitamin C; as did a
professional tennis player who said that his nerves spoilt
his play at crucial points in matches. Damien loved the
game but said that when things got tight, his muscles
tensed and he couldn't control his serve or shots. In his
case, a supplement with calcium and magnesium for
his muscles and pantothenic acid, vitamin C and a B
complex for his tension and adrenals made all the difference. He was grateful for his improved play at crucial
moments, and was later thrilled to report he had more
energy as well.

Your job or your life may involve times of sudden
tension. Having to give a talk; face a classroom of
children; deal with confrontations with neighbours or

customers; cope with social situations when you feel shy or inadequate – all these and situations like them increase your need for the nutrients we have mentioned. If you do not supply them, your adrenal glands will have inadequate resources at times when you need extra energy.

[1] Lewin, S, 1976. *Vitamin C: Its Molecular Biology and Medical Potential*. Academic Press.

[2] ACTH stands for Adreno Cortico Trophic Hormone. It comes from your pituitary gland and stimulates your adrenal glands, just as TSH stimulates your thyroid gland.

Chapter Twelve

Undesirable Energy: Coffee and Other Stimulants

We have already seen that your adrenal glands play a vital role in generating energy. Firstly, they react whenever you are challenged, frightened, nervous, shocked, angry or stressed in any other way. They do this by triggering the release of glucose from glycogen stores into the bloodstream, thus making it available for any cell that needs it for energy. Secondly, even when you are not stressed or challenged, your adrenal glands make sure that your resting blood sugar level remains at normal levels so it is available for the steady work that all the cells do. In Chapter Eleven, we discussed this in some detail, along with the positive, beneficial and nutritional ways in which you can give the adrenals all they need to do their job properly.

There are substances other than nutrients that can stimulate your adrenal glands and give you a lift. One of these is coffee, used by many people to get going in the morning or to stay awake late at night.

I recall a colleague from my days as a geochemist. Let's call him James. He arrived at work one morning looking white and drawn, with a definite case of the jitters. He was clearly very tense and uptight and his first request to the secretary was for a cup of coffee — strong. As luck would have it, we had run out and so, it transpired, had the coffee shop in the building – due to a power cut. He stuck it out for an hour and then announced he had to go out. Half an hour later, he arrived back with a six-pack of cola. An hour later he had drunk the lot and in no time he was back to his normal self.

It transpired that his normal routine was to have several cups of strong black coffee before leaving home in the morning, to get a coke to drink on the train and a cup of coffee on his way into the office building. This morning all these sources had run dry and he was without his usual fix. We had often wondered how James managed to operate so intensely, so fast and so consistently, now we knew. He was high on coffee and cola.

This may seem extreme but it is hardly an exception. If you ask around, you will find that many of the people you know rely heavily on coffee to keep going. They may not recognise this, since coffee is such an accepted part of the daily routine, yet when they have to go without it they notice the difference: they may be not only tired, but irritable, moody and prone to headaches. Many people will say that they cannot give up coffee because they get such bad headaches when they stop drinking it. When I suggest to them that they are drug addicts they look startled, but if you consider a substance that is addictive and behaviour-modifying to be a drug, then that is indeed what coffee is. Other people become addicted to chocolate, some to tea.

Some of the culprit compounds are the methyl xanthines. These include the caffeine in coffee (known chemically as 1,3,7,-tri-methylxanthine), theophylline (1,3,-methylxanthine) found in tea and theobromine (3,7,-dimethylxanthine) found in chocolate. From their chemical names, it is clear that these three compounds are closely related. Of the three, caffeine is the most stimulating, having been described as a 'potent drug, affecting the central nervous system, cardiovascular system, gastrointestinal tract, adrenalin release, muscle contraction'.[1] Probably because caffeine has been so widely used and has such a profound effect on the body, it has been studied extensively.

Coffee affects the central nervous system, as you will know if you have used it to keep alert or stay awake. It may account for some of the hyperactive behaviour in children who have consumed cola and other caffeine-rich drinks. At very high doses, it will cause convulsions, coma and even death. It is estimated that about 10,000 mg will do this. To put that into perspective, the average cup of medium-strength coffee (not a short black which is much stronger) is between 100 mg or 150 mg and so this potentially lethal dose is equivalent to between 70 and 100 cups of coffee.

If this seems like a lot, let me tell you about a man who had such severe heart pains, with no cause the doctors could identify, that he was scheduled for open-heart exploratory surgery. He was drinking up to forty cups of coffee a day and when he stopped, on the advice of a naturopath who was his 'last hope' before the operation, so did the pain. He never did have that exploratory surgery. This is hardly surprising. Light coffee consumption slows the heart down but heavy consumption causes the heart rate to go up and to become irregular. As a result, coffee has an unpredictable effect on blood pressure but usually causes it to rise. It further affects the cardiovascular system by increasing the blood levels of triglycerides and cholesterol, particularly the high-risk form of cholesterol, and even two or three cups a day can do this.

Long term use of coffee for an energy pick-up can result in psychological problems such as nervousness, agitation, disorientation, depression, mood changes, behavioural changes and sleep disorders. These symptoms may be mistaken for anxiety attacks, neurosis or some other disorder and not recognised as resulting from the consumption of coffee.

Coffee is generally thought to increase the production of stomach acid. This is all very well if there is food to be digested at the same time, but can have a harmful effect if coffee is drunk on its own and may even lead to stomach ulcers. However, one separate study has suggested that the reverse occurs and that digestive problems associated with coffee-drinking may result from reduced hydrochloric acid output and incomplete digestion of food. There is yet a third problem in this area. Heavy coffee drinkers often have a weakened sphincter at the base of the oesophagus where it enters the stomach, as a result of which, food can be regurgitated and the rising acid can cause ulcerations in the oesophagus. Further search will doubtless explain these seeming inconsistencies. For our purposes here, it is enough to know that coffee disturbs the normal functioning of your digestive system, particularly in the stomach.

In the long term, although giving you a short-term energy lift, coffee can decrease your ability to generate energy. You need trace nutrients for energy, yet coffee, as a diuretic, is often responsible for the excessive loss of these in the urine. Thus, as time goes on, you need more and more coffee to get the same effect since it is decreasing other avenues of energy production.

Some types of cancer (bladder, pancreas, stomach, colon), miscarriages, possible birth defects and (in at least seven reported cases) death, are the possible adverse side-effects of drinking coffee in large quantities. Ask yourself, is this the way you really want to get energy? If a large amount of coffee can have such dramatic effects, and small amounts obvious and adverse physiological and psychological effects, then why would you want to risk them for just a small amount of energy when there are so many better ways of achieving this goal? Hopefully, by the time you have finished this book you will have found much better ways of generating the energy you want than resorting to coffee.

In closing, it is worth pointing out that the effects of coffee are not entirely the effect of caffeine, though caffeine has often been focused on and labelled as the culprit. In fact, some of the other compounds in coffee may be major causes of some of the problems attributed to coffee. There are many other compounds in coffee that have physiological effects including chlorogenic acid which constitutes between 1.5 and 2.5% of the coffee bean and is known to affect the nervous system.

U.S. figures show that:
Average daily caffeine consumption = 200 mg
30% of the population consumes   = 500 to 600 mg/day
10% of the population consumes more than 1000 mg/day

1 cup of coffee	=	100 to 150 mg of caffeine
1 cup of tea	=	25 to 50 mg of caffeine
1 hot chocolate	=	10 mg of caffeine
1 can of soft drink	=	30 to 60 mg of caffeine
30 gm (1 oz) milk chocolate	=	6 mg of caffeine

What to do

Give up tea, coffee and cola: stop relying on these drinks for energy. Instead, drink herb teas or coffee substitutes. Some herb teas are simply pleasant-tasting, others have added health benefits. Peppermint tea aids digestion, camomile tea is a relaxant, hawthorne tea helps the heart. There are many excellent books available on the benefits of individual herb teas. If you prefer something more like coffee, there are many delicious substitutes made from roasted cereals and other seeds that you can choose from. Dandelion coffee or tea not only tastes good, it is also good for your liver. Since the liver has to work hard in our polluted society where it has to deal with a variety of toxins including social, recreational and medical drugs, pollutants, food additives and so forth, and since a healthy liver is vital for your overall health and energy, this could provide additional benefits (Chapter Eight).

Herb teas are pleasant cold as well as hot. Add ice, a few mint leaves or other herbs, and a slice of lemon. For other cold drinks, turn to fruit juices and mineral water in combinations. Add aloe vera juice and you will be doing your digestive tract a favour.

When you first stop drinking coffee, you may indeed get a headache. This is almost certainly part of your withdrawal symptoms and will not be helped by pain-killers. The only things that will help is a cup of coffee – the hair of the dog. If you truly cannot stand the pain, then have a tiny amount of coffee, just enough to get you through this time. It will delay and prolong the process but this is up to you. If you can handle the headache, then live with it. In a few hours, a few days at the most – depending on how addicted you are, how much coffee you have been drinking and how your body has reacted – it will be gone, and gone for good, provided you don't become a coffee addict all over again.

Other Stimulants and your Energy

Similarly, other stimulants may seem to give you the energy you want but are only a short-term solution. The effect does not last. Nor have you solved the fundamental problem, the cause of your lack of energy. Put the ideas of this book into practice and you will be changing things at the grass-roots level. Once you have done that, you won't need, and probably won't want, stimulants. Not only do stimulants not provide a real solution, they can cause problems of their own.

Some people turn to alcohol for a new lease of life. This produces negative effects, apart from those of getting drunk. Alcohol puts a toxic strain on the liver. The alcohol is converted into a variety of other chemicals that are harmful and it is the job of your liver to deal with these. It needs more of the B group vitamins, plus lecithin. It also needs methionine, the sulphur-containing amino acid found in highest quantities in eggs, that causes the dreadful smell of bad eggs as hydrogen sulphide and other sulphur compounds are formed. Your liver will also need all the antioxidants it can get to deal with the various free radicals that are formed. In addition, as we have seen, alcohol can interfere with your absorption of vitamin B12 and a lack of this vitamin can cause anaemia and fatigue, the very problem you are trying to solve. Alcohol is also a diuretic.

All this should convince you that alcohol does not give you energy, that, ultimately it depletes your body of vital nutrients which would generate energy, and strains and damages the liver just when you need all the help you can get from your liver in dealing with toxins and performing the hundreds of reactions for which it is responsible.

Marijuana may make you feel better, but it certainly doesn't help provide more energy. It may help to obliterate the problem, at least for a while, but it won't help you to get anything done. Cocaine may seem to be providing more help but much the same is true for this drug as for alcohol. Any apparent help is shortlived, the toxic side-effects are longlived, there is the problem of addiction and you have not dealt with the fundamental cause of your problem.

References

Bolton S., Null G., Pressman A.H., 'Caffeine, its effect, uses and abuses', *Applied Nutrition*, 33, 1981, p.35.

See also Xandria Williams 'What's wrong with coffee and chocolate and cola and . . .', *Australian Wellbeing* No.13, 1986, p. 29.

PART III

Using Up More Energy or Increasing the Need for Energy

There are many health problems and diseases that deplete your energy levels. Tiredness may be one of the first overt symptoms that occurs, yet not be the primary problem of itself, but rather a hint that something deeper is wrong. For this reason, it is unwise to ignore tiredness or to simply put it down to increasing age and having too much to do.

Emotions can cause exhaustion, even pleasurable ones. Negative or unplesasant emotions can certainly leave you feeling tired and drained.

We shall assume that you have already worked through Parts I and II of this book and have attended to all that is indicated there. If you have done that and are still tired, there may indeed be some other health problem that needs attention. You should investigate this possibility and endeavour to find its source.

You may be under physical or emotional stress. Stress can be exhausting and we shall look, in this section, on the effect it can have on your body and energy level. Your blood sugar level may be erratic. When it is low you will inevitably run short of energy and feel tired. If it falls to below normal levels with abnormal ease and frequency, you are probably suffering from hypoglycae-

mia, which warrants attention, both for itself and in case
it should lead on to diabetes.

Your heart is of vital importance in supplying blood
and oxygen to the cells throughout your body. If this is
not done correctly, you will not be able to 'burn up' the
food you eat as fuel and so will be unable to generate
energy. Heart problems can lead to tiredness.

Similarly, respiratory problems, from relatively minor
ones such as hay fever (which can be exhausting) and
sinus problems, to major ones like asthma and emphysema can lead to inadequate oxygen supply and reduced
energy levels. In fact, the problem is twofold. The disease
itself is exhausting *and* it interferes with normal energy
production.

For the past few years, thrush, caused by an overgrowth of *candida albicans*, has been widely recognised
as a major health problem and one that often goes undiagnosed. It creates a wide spectrum of symptoms, many
of them mimicking other health problems, and most of
them being vague and difficult to assess or define. High
on this list are mood changes and generalised fatigue.
Organisms other than *candida albicans* can also create
fatigue, from parasites to infections related to a variety
of bacteria and viruses.

Like thrush and hypoglycaemia, the significance of
allergies is often missed. Yet for the past fifty or more
years it has been obvious to people who specialise in
this field that the effects of allergies are pervasive,
exhausting and frequently go unrecognised.

Being overweight can be exhausting. If you are one
stone (or nearly seven kilo) overweight, it is like carrying
an equivalent weight – perhaps a very heavy shopping
bag – around with you. If you are three stone (or twenty
kilos) overweight, it is like carrying a large, heavy suitcase around with you (equivalent to the weight you can
take on an overseas flight). The effort may not seem so

great when the weight is distributed all over you as when it is carried in one hand as a bag or suitcase, but the stress on your body is there none the less. Rough estimates suggest that there are hundreds of miles of blood vessels in each pound of flesh. Think of the extra work that your heart and circulation system have to do each time you gain a pound.

These in particular and other health problems in general can all contribute to low energy levels and should be corrected as part of your drive to get your energy back.

The following chapters are not intended to offer a complete treatment programme for each of the disease states that can lead to fatigue and loss of energy. It should be obvious that almost any health problem can lead to fatigue and there is not room to discuss them all in this book. If any of the disease states mentioned above are overtly present, specific therapy by a fully-qualified health-care professional is probably indicated. However, it is possible for there to be mild indications of the problems discussed, in which case the treatments indicated in this section could be preventative. They may stop the disease developing or slow down its progress and will almost certainly improve your energy.

Critical care may be needed for many of these conditions if they become severe. Hypoglycaemia, for instance, may develop into diabetes. That, like asthma and heart disease, may require serious medical attention. However, improved nutrition will also certainly help in conjunction with whatever else is done. The treatments indicated in this section can be followed alongside any other treatments you may be receiving already, and you may well be surprised at the increase in energy that results.

Finally, it is worth pointing out that there are several factors that are common to many of the health problems described in this section. Firstly, they all lead to fatigue; secondly, they can all be treated in large part by diet and lifestyle modification and by the use of nutritional supplements. A third factor, however, is of more concern: namely, that the majority of them are not problems that are commonly looked for, detected, recognised or treated by conventional medicine. Many mainstream doctors fail to pay attention to the problems of stress-induced under-nutrition, thrush, hypoglycaemia or food sensitivities and clinical ecology (the broader concept of allergies used by natural therapists). For this reason, the cause and hence the solution to your tiredness may well have been missed. Sinus problems and asthma can often be resolved to a significant extent, as we shall see, by proper attention to allergies – food allergies as well as environmental allergies. On the other hand, heart problems in their broadest context are widely recognised as having a basis in food and lifestyle.

Chronic Fatigue Syndrome

We shall be dealing with Chronic Fatigue Syndrome more fully in Part IV, but is worth mentioning here that many of the topics we discuss in this section are also relevant to the treatment for CFS. For instance, reduced immune function, the presence of a variety of organisms, including *candida*, toxins, hypoglycaemia and allergies may all play a significant role in both the development of and the treatment of CFS and so mention will be made of CFS from time to time as we go through this section.

Chapter Thirteen

Emotions

Emotions can be exhausting. Happy emotions, excitement, joy, anticipation – these and other positive emotions, while feeling wonderful, can also be tiring. No one can live at a fever-pitch of excitement for long. However the dramatic phase soon passes and you can generally relax and enjoy the quieter positive emotions.

Negative emotions, on the other hand, can cause both short-term and prolonged fatigue. They can cause fatigue in themselves. If the situations behind these emotions are not resolved, you have a prolonged emotional experience that depletes your energy reserves on a long-term basis.

This is not the place to discuss how to overcome and resolve these negative emotions, although countless books have been written on the subjects.[1] There is a great deal you can do to handle these emotions and resolve the issues involved. Once you make a start, you may be surprised at how easy it is to make the necessary changes. However, what we are concerned with here is how these emotions affect your energy at the physical level.

When you experience any of these negative emotions the impact is felt, almost immediately, in your digestive tract. Perhaps you have to give a speech, or face someone who makes you nervous. You've probably had the experience of feeling you simply had to go to the toilet, and not once but several times. If you are frightened, your mouth goes dry and it is difficult to chew or swallow. In fact the whole of your digestive tract 'goes dry' and it is equally difficult for food to be passed along the entire length of it. When you have been sad or upset you have probably experienced a loss of appetite, at least temporarily. These are short-term effects of your emotions on your body, particularly on your digestive system.

There are long-term effects too. Irritability, anger and stress are classically associated with stomach and duodenal ulcers. Long-term stress leads to stasis and constipation and this in turn leads to the production of toxins that are absorbed into your body and further deplete your resources. These toxins can leave you feeling not only tired and lacking in initiative but also feeling as if you are trying to think in a fog.

When these emotions occur and generate stress, the sympathetic nervous system and related hormone systems come into play, triggering the fight or flight mechanism. We have mentioned this already (Chapter Eleven). When this happens, your body is alert to things in the outside world and the digestive process slows down almost entirely. If you continue to feel these emotions on a long-term basis and your digestive system consequently remains below its normal level of function, you will find it is very difficult to digest your meals properly. The consequence of this, of course, is that you do not break the foods down properly, you do not absorb them and you become undernourished and so even more tired. (See Chapter Three.)

The situation is worsened if your emotional state leaves you indifferent to the food you eat. You may say you are so cross you can't be bothered with cooking, or you are too depressed to make the effort to go out and shop. You may be so focused on whatever it is that is worrying you that you grab whatever snack is available. Almost certainly this will not give you the nutrients you need, and yet ironically, while you are stressed in this way you have an *increased* need for nutrients, just at the time when you are neither giving them to yourself nor digesting your food properly.

If you take the next step and tell yourself you are so unhappy you deserve something nice to eat as compensation you could be in even more trouble from a nutritional standpoint. It is unlikely that such a 'treat' will involve a raw carrot, a salad or some fresh fruit. It is much more likely to be a bar of chocolate, some ice-cream or some other equally non-nutritious food.

What to do

However stressed you are, make the decision that your health is of paramount importance. Recognise that while you are stressed, your nutrition is even more important than when you are relaxed and happy. Plan to buy and cook nutritious meals and allow yourself the time to relax and eat them. If your car ran out of petrol, you would not kick it and complain that it was useless or give it a new coat of paint to make it look good. You would feed it properly, topping it up with the correct petrol, oil and water. Your body also needs the appropriate fuel, yet people often seem to forget this. It's as if they think of food as something simply to provide flavours and a feeling of fullness, and ignore or are unaware of all the other roles it plays – its crucial nutritional value, and the reactions that have to go on inside your body for you to function at your best.

Once you have read the rest of this section on the way energy is generated in your body, you will be more aware of the details than you were before. Perhaps for you this is a first step in the direction of better nourishment, no matter what mood you are in.

Even assuming you do have a good meal on the table while you have all these negative emotions running around, there can still be problems unless you can learn to relax. Even if you cannot resolve the emotions, at least make a conscious effort to relax physically. Sit down. You cannot digest a meal properly if you are on the move. Sit up straight. If you slouch over and cramp up your digestive organs you cannot expect them to work properly. Put your shoulders back, and down. Relax your abdominal muscles, let your stomach and abdomen 'hang out'. Take some deep breaths and promise yourself not to talk about anything worrying while you are eating.

For many people, mealtimes are associated with tension even if the rest of the day is reasonably calm. If this is part of your problem, then getting some help, digging up the buried issues and releasing them may be what it takes to improve your digestion, improve your health and give you more energy.

There are many practitioners who can help you with this. Find someone who specialises in Neurolinguistic Programming (NLP): they should be able to help you resolve and release the emotions within a few sessions and without trauma. After all, you are trying to get your energy back – you do not want to be going through the, sometimes debilitating, process of reliving past problems or stirring up old memories and issues. NLP offers ways of resolving the situations without having to do this.

[1] Xandria Williams, *Stress – recognise and resolve*, Charles Letts & Co. Ltd, 1993.
Xandria Williams, *Beating the Blues*, Cedar, 1995.

Chapter Fourteen

Stress

The word 'stress' is so much a part of our current vocabulary that you might be forgiven for thinking it has been with us, as a word with its current usage, for a long time. This is not so. Until relatively recently people would talk about being worried (over money), over-worked, harried (by the demands of their boss), anxious (about their children). They were specific about the emotion they were feeling and about the reason they were feeling it. 'Stress' as a catch-all term was rarely used, certainly not in the way in which it is today.

Similarly, in the physical sense, it was not used in the way we use it now. The turning-point came with the work of Hans Selye. Selye observed that when any health problem occurred there were certain reactions that always occurred within the body. These were common to all outside challenges, all illnesses, no matter what their nature and no matter what the ultimate health consequence. He recognised this as a core process, the body's response to perturbation, no matter of what type. He identified, recognised and described three stages to this core process and called the totality the stress response.

Stage I is the Alarm Stage. This is your initial response to an alarm signal – the roar of a lion, the sight of a car coming straight at you, the effect of chemical toxins, an unpleasant confrontation, or the sudden thought of a problem, anxiety or fear. During this stage, there is a rush of adrenalin from your adrenal glands into the bloodstream and this adrenalin alerts your cells to the imminent need for action. You will have felt this yourself many times. You may even have labelled it, correctly, as a rush of adrenalin. This first sequence of reactions closes down your digestive system and your urinary system, as we have already seen, and pumps blood to your muscles. This stage leads to the acute and often obvious symptoms of immediate and reactive stress.

Stage II is the Adaptive Stage. It is not possible for you to stay in the Alarm Stage for any length of time. You know yourself how you eventually adapt to whatever stress is applied. Your body and your emotions are amazingly resilient. No matter how bad the situation, you learn, at least for a while, to adapt and to handle things. When you get bad news there may be initial panic followed by a relative calm as you learn to deal with the problem. No one likes the fear of war, but when in the thick of it you learn to adapt and to live with it. You may hate having an in-law to live with you, but eventually you adapt and cope. So does your body. It moves from the Alarm Stage into this Adaptive Stage

During this stage, which can be prolonged, the amount of adrenalin circulating in your blood is reduced and other hormones are released instead. Other chemical changes also occur. Your body needs more nutrients but, since it probably won't get them, it learns to cope, at least temporarily, and comes to terms with health problems for a while. You may not, during this stage, be full of energy, you may not be vibrantly healthy, but you have learnt to adapt and cope.

Let's take an example. Initially, allergens and toxins may have caused an acute reaction. Eventually the allergen reaction is 'masked' and the body adapts; the effects of the toxins are dealt with at the cellular level and you become used to the symptoms and ignore them. You may have stopped showing the immediate symptoms and instead have become chemically addicted both to the toxins and the allergens. The result is to reduce your overall health and energy. It may be like trying to work through a mental fog. You may have days when you drag yourself around. You *have* adapted but you *are* tired.

It is almost certain that you are not consciously aware of this adaptation. You may know you have been under stress or subjected to additional strains, emotional or physical, but you have kept going. You may even be patting yourself on the back for your ability to cope, to keep going, even when you are not feeling terrific. Yet there is an ongoing price to pay. You are drawing on cellular reserves – living on capital. Because there are no obvious and clear cut symptoms and because you have good days and days that are not so good, it is probable that on the good days you increase the amount that you do, to make use of the sudden resurgence of energy you seem to have. Unfortunately, in this way you are subjecting your system to further stress and you will eventually reach the limit of its capacity to cope.

Ideally, this Adaptive Stage should be used for recuperation and recovery. It should not be taken as an indication that you can handle the imposed stresses and continue to keep going under their weight. If you do not use this stage constructively, you will find yourself in the final stage.

You will enter Stage III, the Exhaustion Stage. When you reach the end of your resources and your capacity to cope (the end of Stage II), alarm bells are set off throughout your body, just as they were in the initial Alarm Stage. However, whereas when it happened initially you had a reserve of resources to deal with the situation, now there are no more reserves. You cannot pump out the adrenalin and leap into action as you did in Stage I. You are worn out. Your organs and systems, such as the digestive system, the liver, the adrenal glands, your nervous system, the immune system, are worn out. They have nothing more to give.

As a result of entering the Exhaustion Stage, a number of significant health problems become obvious, if they have not already done so. Digestive problems involving both the digestive tract itself and the liver occur. In your nervous system, the stress leads to increased anxiety, confusion, dizziness, inability to concentrate, depression, lack of motivation and other mood changes. You are aware you are not coping and this worries you and further increases the stresses you feel. The weakened immune system may lead to increased infections or to auto-immune diseases such as rheumatism and other muscular and skeletal aches and pains. You may develop eczema, hay fever or asthma.

You will certainly feel tired and probably exhausted. You may, in fact, have just entered into the situation described as Chronic Fatigue Syndrome. This is unfortunate, to say the least. It is very much easier to fix the problem in either the Alarm Stage (Stage I) or the Adaptive Stage (Stage II) than it is once you have reached the Exhaustion Stage (Stage III). If you are tired and feel you are heading in this direction, near the end of your tether, the end of your ability to cope and thus the end of the Adaptive Stage, then do something *now*, before you reach exhaustion.

It is all too easy to put this off. It is all too easy, on your bad and tired days, to say you are too tired to make the effort to shop and prepare better food, too tired to make the effort to take supplements, too tired to organise a water purifier, too tired to take proper care of yourself. You tell yourself you are too tired to initiate whatever changes are necessary in your life. All you have the energy for, you may be telling yourself, is the bare essentials for survival before you collapse into bed.

On the other hand, on your good days, you may be so pleased that you do have some energy that you rush to do all the chores you have been putting off on the bad days when you were exhausted. In this way you are piling more stresses on yourself, further depleting your reserves and rushing headlong towards the Exhaustion Stage. Stop. Don't do this. Do something to solve the problem, now, before it is too late. There are no prizes for being heroic, for compromising your health until you reach the point of being of no use to anyone, least of all to yourself. Make a decision not to go on 'putting up' with a situation.

If there are people who annoy you, work on your response. Your anger is harming you, not them. If your workload is too great, make changes. If you haven't had a holiday for years, take one. If you have to work in a polluted environment, do all you can to cut down on the level of pollution, then protect yourself with a mask, protective clothing, by moving further from computer screens, or whatever else is possible.

Remember, the Stress Response is meant to be a useful way for your body to handle whatever challenges it has to cope with. In the ideal situation, the Alarm Reaction should alert you to the problem. The Adaptive Stage should then give you time and resources to cope calmly. Ideally, you should then relax and restore your reserves so that next time an emergency hits you can start all over again. It is unwise to assume that you can remain in this Adaptive Stage for ever without taking stock and replacing your depleted resources.

What To Do

There are all sorts of ways of handling stress. Factors
that distress you emotionally and mentally can be dealt
with and this has been covered elsewhere.[1] Factors that
stress you physically should be avoided or dealt with
constructively. Do all you can to minimise the stresses
in your life that have a negative effect – which is probably most of them. Then increase your body's ability to
handle the stresses that do occur by giving it proper
nutrition and, where necessary, supplements. Make
many of the positive changes indicated in this book.

[1] Xandria Williams, *Stress – recognise and resolve*. Charles Letts and Co
Ltd, 1993.

Chapter Fifteen

Hypoglycaemia

Twenty years ago, I could write that 'In patients who are tired or who are cross, irritable and feel they can't cope with what they have to do in the day, hypoglycaemia is frequently part of the problem. Almost as frequently it goes unrecognised. If you see a naturopath there is a chance they will detect it. If you see a doctor there is almost no chance at all since on the whole doctors don't believe it exists or that, if it does, it is a transient part of the diabetes pattern and of little or no concern to people who are not diabetic.' Things have changed slightly today, but only slightly. It is even more readily recognised by naturopaths and, thankfully, there are also some doctors who are recognising it and the untold misery it can cause. Yet even now the majority of doctors give it little credence and all too often the symptoms go unrecognised.

You may be suffering from bouts of sudden energy-loss accompanied by several symptoms which we will consider shortly — you may in fact be hypoglycaemic — yet your doctor may still tell you to 'buck up', to be 'grateful for what you have' — such as the children who are making so many demands on you, the successful husband for whom you have to do so much entertaining, or the exciting job that requires you to work overtime. Alternatively you may be led to understand, however

subtly, that it is 'all in your head' and find yourself being
told 'go home and rest, you'll soon be fine'. You may
get the impression they think you are making a fuss
about nothing, mountains out of molehills, that you are
imagining things, or seeking attention. You may even be
given an anti-depressant or a tranquiliser to soothe you
and stop you worrying.

Hypoglycaemia, however, has a distinct symptom pattern, a set of physiological events that explain the symptoms, and a workable treatment programme. If this is
your problem, you should learn to understand it for this
leads to the ability to treat and, eventually, solve the
problem.

Normal Blood Sugar Patterns

The word 'hypoglycaemia' means low (*hypo*) sugar (*glyc*)
in the blood (*aemia*). To understand what is happening
when your blood sugar level falls and your energy falls
with it, you need to understand your normal blood sugar
pattern.

Under normal, fasting conditions (periods when you
have not eaten for a few hours), your blood glucose level
lies within certain limits (60–110mg/100 ml or 3.5–6.0
mmol/l) considered to be the normal range. When you
eat a meal, this rises as you absorb glucose from the
food, then falls back to normal. If it ever falls significantly below normal, this is the condition of hypoglycaemia.

When you eat a meal, it will almost inevitably contain
some carbohydrate, from grains, fruit, vegetables or
sugar. Ideally, of course, this carbohydrate should be
from complex carbohydrates such as the starches from
grains and vegetables. As we saw in Chapter Three,
these starch molecules are then gradually stripped of
one glucose molecule after another and these in turn

start a steady trickle of glucose into the bloodstream. This glucose-rich blood travels throughout the body. In response to the raised blood sugar level, your pancreas pumps out insulin which encourages the glucose to enter cells and thus the blood sugar level remains only slightly high, until it eventually returns to normal when the absorption of food is complete and your body returns to the fasting state.

If you eat refined carbohydrates, such as white flour, white pasta or white rice, then the starch breaks down much faster and the blood sugar level rises much higher before the insulin gets to work and starts pushing the glucose into the cells and can bring it back down to normal. There may even be an oversupply of insulin, since the pancreas cannot be aware of when this sugar flood is likely to stop. This excess insulin may push too much glucose into the cells and your blood sugar level may fall a little below normal. Other hormones then become active, including glucagon from the pancreas and adrenalin from the adrenal glands. Their job is to mobilise glucose from inside the cells and send it back out into the bloodstream to keep your blood sugar levels up to the normal level.

When you eat refined carbohydrates such as sugar, honey, fructose and glucose, little digestion is required and so these are absorbed extremely rapidly into your bloodstream and there is a very rapid rise in blood sugar level. As a result, an equivalently high output of insulin occurs, plus some overkill and the blood sugar levels can fall even further on the rebound. If you are still relatively healthy, glucagon and adrenalin will yet again rush out and push the blood sugar level up, just as before, possibly even overreacting, in which case more insulin could be needed, and the cycle repeats until it all settles back to normal.

If, however, you have been eating a diet low in the B

group vitamins (such as occurs when you eat white flour, white rice or sugar) your adrenal glands are probably too tired to do their job properly (see Chapter Eleven). When your blood sugar level then falls, it is allowed to fall too far and to remain low for too long, and as a result the unpleasant symptoms occur for a while, until the various hormones belatedly push your blood sugar level up again. Initially this may occur only occasionally, or only when you eat a large amount of sugar. In time you may find that this scenario occurs more and more frequently and the symptoms are more severe and last longer.

To get this into perspective, let's consider the quantities involved, using round figures. The total volume of blood in someone weighing around 70 kg is usually about five-and-a-half litres (5500 cc). The red cells take up about two litres (2000 cc), so the volume of the plasma, the blood liquid, is about three-and-a-half litres (3500 cc). If this, for argument's sake, contains about 80 mg of glucose per 100 ml, then the total amount of glucose in the plasma is $80/100 \times 3500$ mg = 2800 mg, or nearly 3 gm. This would easily fit onto the average size teaspoon and lie relatively flat.

What happens when you eat a candy bar of, say 60 g or two ounces that is fifty per cent sugar (and many are closer to one hundred per cent sugar)? You probably eat it relatively fast. There is virtually no digesting to do: it simply goes straight down the tubes to the small intestine where it crosses over into the bloodstream. Thus there is a sudden arrival of 30 g or more of glucose delivered into a bloodstream that normally contains only 3 g in total – a tenfold overload. As soon as the first molecules arrive and your blood sugar level starts to rise, the pancreas pumps out insulin and tries to drive it into the cells, but this amount of sugar is still a huge overload on the system. All this takes only a few minutes to happen.

On the other hand, if you eat a plateful of porridge, consisting of, say 60 g of dry rolled oats, which in turn contains about 40 g of carbohydrate, this takes about four hours to be completely digested and for the large starch molecules to be broken down fully to individual glucose molecules and absorbed into the bloodstream. This means that there is no sudden surge of glucose entering the bloodstream, but rather, a steady trickle over four hours.

If we assume it takes you three minutes to eat the candy bar, it gives you a sugar hit of 30 mg of glucose into the bloodstream in that time, or approximately 10 g of glucose a minute. This overwhelms the glucose-handling system. The porridge, on the other hand, gives you 40 g of sugar over four hours, or 10 g an hour. This is one-sixtieth of the delivery rate and a manageable amount that the glucose-handling system can deal with.

There is clearly a vast difference in the way your body experiences the result of eating complex and unrefined carbohydrates on the one hand, and highly-refined carbohydrates or sugars on the other. It is now time to find out what symptoms can result when your body can no longer handle these overloads to your blood sugar level.

Low Blood Sugar Level Symptoms

When cells need energy, especially when they need it in a hurry, their first choice is the glucose in your bloodstream. However, most of them are readily able to take up fatty acids for energy if your blood glucose level is low. An exception to this is your brain. Your brain cells are heavily reliant on glucose for energy. Only when you fast for several days and your blood glucose is gradually used up do your brain cells convert, slowly, to using fatty acids for energy instead of glucose. Many of the unpleasant symptoms that can occur at the start of a fast are due to this drop in energy in the brain as the blood sugar level falls and before the switch to fatty acid metabolism has occurred.

If your blood sugar level falls as part of the aftermath of a meal or snack rich in sugars or refined carbohydrates, then a variety of unpleasant symptoms may result. The physical symptoms can include weakness and low energy, a hollow feeling in the abdomen ('stomach'), hunger and nausea, shaking in the hands and throughout the body, headache, dizziness and palpitations. The mental symptoms can include irritability, anxiety, and panic attacks, mood swings, sudden bursts of temper followed by tears and even quite marked changes in personality. You may also experience an overwhelming desire to eat – anything – to get rid of the symptoms. This is when your diet and all your good intentions go out of the window and you eat as much as you can as fast as you can.

These symptoms may send you out searching for a bar of chocolate, some sweets, biscuits or cake, even a tub of ice-cream. As you stuff yourself full of these, nothing much happens to start with. This is because it takes time for this sugar to reach first your bloodstream and then your cells. In real terms it is not long, but it may seem like an age when you are feeling dreadful. You probably go on eating until you finally feel better, but by then you have overshot the mark and your blood sugar level is on its way up again to a high point, insulin is being pumped out trying to rush your blood glucose level back down again, it overshoots, and your blood sugar level falls to below the normal level ... and the cycle is starting all over again.

Using sugar to solve a low blood glucose problem

may seem logical but in fact is a disastrous mistake. Each sugar 'solution' provides the cause of the next 'high' and so the next 'low' and the next group of symptoms.

The use of alcohol is no better. Some people try to solve an energy slump with, for instance, a stiff whisky. You will often see them down the full glass so fast you wonder if they have even tasted it. Then they may drink nothing for thirty to sixty minutes. It is probable that their blood sugar level has risen and they feel fine, then it falls again and they hit the next glass.

> *David was a typical case in point. He would come home from work, tired and stressed, drink a stiff whisky poured for him by his wife, then relax, play with the children and chat. After about half an hour he would pour himself a second drink and joke with her about not keeping up. About two drinks later, they would sit down to dinner, by which time he was rarely hungry. A couple more drinks after dinner and he would be asleep. His wife, who had come to see me, said it was destroying their marriage. His moods would yo-yo up and down when he first came home and by nine or ten o'clock he was too drunk for sensible conversation. What she couldn't understand, she said, was why he drank so fast. He didn't seem to enjoy the drinks, simply threw them back like medication, as indeed they were. When I eventually saw David and explained about the blood sugar pattern he agreed to take a nutritional supplement and to eat sensible snacks (raw nuts in his case) through the after-noon and thus prevent the hypo he attempted to 'solve' with his drinking. As a result, they were able to have a couple of leisurely drinks before dinner and enjoy the rest of their evening together.*

As in David's case, the cycle of low blood sugar, a drink to raise it and feel good, then a hypo followed by the next drink, repeats until, as the drinks get closer and closer together, you get drunk and fall asleep. The best solution to hypoglycaemia is always to find the cause and prevent the original 'hypo'.

Causes of Hypoglycaemia

An obvious cause of hypoglycaemia is eating too much sugar and too many refined carbohydrates, so these should be eliminated from the diet. This will not only remove one of the triggering factors to hypoglycaemia, it will also, almost certainly, improve the nutritional content of your diet.

A secondary cause is a lack of the nutrients for the proper metabolism of glucose. These include the B group vitamins, and several trace minerals, including zinc, magnesium and manganese. Your diet should be changed to include foods rich in these nutrients. This will happen automatically if you change from eating white flour to wholemeal, from white rice to brown rice and from eating sugar to eating fruits and more whole grains. You should also add these nutrients in supplement form as you have a deficit to replace and, as we have seen (Chapter Two), even the best of diets will not provide ample sufficiency.

A third cause is skipping meals. Missing meals allows your blood sugar level to fall. Instead of allowing large gaps between meals, you should eat several small and nutritious meals at intervals of about two hours apart, throughout the day. Working hard for long periods without taking a rest, and stress, are all possible contributing factors to hypoglycaemia and you should make the appropriate changes there too. Another possible cause of hypoglycaemia is allergies which we will discuss later (see Chapter Eighteen).

I recall a patient, in my early days in practice, who came to see me in a filthy temper. We'll call her Susan. She had been kept waiting for all of five minutes in the waiting-room but you would have thought it was five hours. She marched into my office, almost refused to sit down, and spent the next five minutes angrily telling me how I should be running my practice and complaining of what was wrong in the world in general and her world in particular.

Eventually she calmed down and I saw a dumpy woman in her mid-thirties. She was plain, overweight, with a pasty complexion, pimples and lank untidy hair. The problem, she told me, was her pimples, followed a close second by her weight. It turned out that she knew what to eat, namely fresh fruit and vegetables, a high-fibre diet low in fat and with sufficient protein, etc., and that she would stick at that for several days in a row. Then she'd suddenly get fed up with the whole thing, get a craving for something sweet and go off and eat a packet of biscuits. She'd then have a few days on this sugar-rich diet and, I surmised, her blood sugar levels would go haywire. Her moods would be all over the place and her friends would run for cover. She wanted to meet someone and get married but, as she said in her more clear-sighted state of relaxation, no one could stand her for long. After a couple of satisfactory dates, something would usually happen by the third one and she'd throw a tantrum and the man would depart.

I sent her for a glucose-tolerance test, which involved drinking a glass of water with 100 g of glucose and taking blood sugar readings beforehand and every thirty minutes afterwards for a period of six hours. During the test she had a major 'hypo', threw a huge tantrum and, since fortunately her blood sugar level was being measured right in the middle of it, saw that this occurred at the same time as a slump in the level. This convinced her of the cause of the problem and she was willing to work at the solution.

Even though she knew what to eat, and would even eat wisely for a few days, she was clearly eating the wrong foods most of the time and getting both too much sugar and not enough vitamins and minerals. After the test had been done, she started on a treatment programme (described later) and became a lot more relaxed. Most of the time she was able to stick to the foods she knew were good for her health, for her skin and for her energy. She was also able to avoid the sugar binges. As a result, most of the time she was able to keep her energy and moods stable. She stopped gaining weight, even lost a little occasionally, her skin improved slightly and her friends said she was a lot easier to be with. However, from time to time she would still plunge back into the old pattern. She said it was a bit like living on a knife-edge, never quite knowing when she would fall off.

Hypoglycaemia is, in a sense, not a problem in itself but is rather the symptom of some other, deeper problem. The possibilities include adrenal exhaustion, undernutrition, stress and allergies.

In Susan's case I suspected that allergies were part of her problem. The tests confirmed this and showed her to be allergic to wheat, peanuts and chocolate. When the amount of these foods in her normal diet increased, her blood sugar level eventually became particularly erratic until such time as the plunge got the better of her self-control and she went into a hypo and an eating binge. Since the eating binge included these three foods in the form of cakes, biscuits, peanut butter, chocolate and (chocolate) ice-cream, the binge sent her blood sugar levels gyrating like a rollercoaster and it would take her several days to restore her equilibrium.

Once she cut these allergenic foods totally out of her

diet, she said everything became much easier. She no longer felt she was living on a knife-edge. She was able to relax, eat the foods she knew were good for her, avoid the hypos and so avoid the binges. As a result, she lost weight and her skin improved dramatically, and so did her moods. Her energy went up and stayed up. Best of all, some years later, she phoned to tell me she had married and had a child. The most profound statement she made was to the effect that she had gone through ten years of hell which could have been avoided had those same simple dietary changes been made earlier.

The Test

A six-hour glucose tolerance test (GTT), with blood sugar levels measured every thirty minutes, will soon tell you whether or not you are hypoglycaemic. But be warned: many people will do a test that is not so thorough yet still purport to be able to assure you that hypoglycaemia is not your problem. The consequences of missing this diagnosis are too great for you to take this risk, as Susan found out. Before you rule out hypoglycaemia as the cause of your lack of energy and other health problems, be sure that you have had a thorough test done.

Some people will only take your blood sugar level every hour instead of every half-hour. Yet it is common to find that the fall in blood sugar level, to a point that would, if detected, indicate hypoglycaemia, and its return to normal, can happen within the sixty-minute period between two tests. Other practitioners will only continue the tests for three hours, not six. This too is inadequate.

Take the following example of someone who had had the complete test done covering a six-hour period with samples taken every half-hour. Her results were as follows:

At the start of the test her blood sugar level was **85** mg (before the glass of glucose and water), rising to 110, **170**, 150, **140**, 125, **100**, 60, **80**, 90 and finally back to 85mg.

- On the basis of the complete set of results, she was definitely hypoglycaemic, as shown by the drop to 60 mg and the slow recovery to 80 mg before returning to her normal of 85 mg.
- On the basis of the results taken at hourly intervals (the results marked in bold), she would have been told that her results were normal. The result of 60 that would have shown that hypoglycaemia *was* part of her problem would have been missed and the result of 80 would have been considered insignificant on its own.
- On the basis of the short test, for three hours only, whether at hourly or half-hourly intervals, her final reading would have been 100 mg and the hypoglycaemic section of the curve would have been missed
- Finally, it is important that you record your symptoms at every half-hour point, particularly in relation to such things as headaches, dizziness, feeling faint, shaky, irritable, nervous and so forth. In the above example she experienced a number of unpleasant symptoms at the 60 mg point including tiredness, headache, the 'shakes', irritability or some other mood change.

So make sure that, if you have the test done, it lasts for six hours, measurements are taken every thirty minutes and that you are asked to fill out a symptom questionnaire with every measurement.

Simple Treatment

This simple test will show you whether or not you are hypoglycaemic. However, the symptoms are often sufficient to alert you. If you wish to avoid having the test done, or can find no one who will do it as described above but suspect from your symptoms that you are hypoglycaemic, then try the treatment and see if it works. If it does, hypoglycaemia was probably the problem.

You have little to lose by trying this, since the treatment will almost certainly result in an improvement to your diet and supplements and so to improved general health. If the treatment does not solve the problem, your situation is less clear. Your energy slumps could have a totally different cause or there could be, in addition to hypoglycaemia, other confounding factors, as in Susan's case, that also have to be resolved.

As part of the treatment, it is important that you give up sugars altogether. You will find this easier to do if you have a high intake of the B group vitamins, especially vitamin B1. You should then eat small frequent meals at regular intervals throughout the day, ensuring you don't ever let your blood sugar level fall. These meals should not be the usual snack foods. Although they are only small snacks, it is essential that they are as nutritious as if they were your main meal of the day. In fact, many people do make one main meal but they eat it in three sections over six hours. Eat complex carbohydrates (starches and not sugars) and use wholemeal not refined grains (wholemeal as opposed to white flour) supplements of all the B group vitamins, especially B1, B3 and B5, vitamin C and a trace mineral supplement rich in chromium, magnesium, manganese and zinc.

Keep in mind that the lack of energy associated with hypoglycaemia is likely to be episodic. It will alternate with periods when you feel perfectly normal and seem to have lots of energy. The energy-drop and associated symptoms may come after meals, after eating sweets, or after a long time without food. Your symptoms will probably improve when you eat.

Even if you do feel you can cope with the hypoglycaemia, now that you know what it is, you should not continue to ignore it. In itself it may be a relatively insignificant problem. However, it can be the step that leads on to diabetes. If you continue on the sugar binges each time your energy level falls, a time may come when not only are your adrenal glands exhausted and unable to shore up the falling blood sugar level, but your pancreas may become exhausted too. Your pancreas may be unable to continue pumping out the large amounts of insulin required by your high sugar intake. Your blood sugar level then remains high and you have become diabetic. There is argument over this point: some doctors feel that a high consumption of sugar is not a precursor to diabetes, but many others think that it is or that, at the very least, the high sugar intake can be a contributing factor.

Both for itself and for what it can lead to, hypoglycaemia should be detected, treated and cured. Clearly, this will not only help to improve the hypoglycaemia; it will also lead to better health in general and increased energy.

Chapter Sixteen

Thrush

Candida albicans is a yeast or mould which is present in everyone soon after birth. This may not have been so thousands of years ago, but nowadays most babies have some *candida albicans* organisms present within their digestive tract within months of their birth. It thrives in warm, dark and wet places and so does very well throughout the length of the digestive tract and in the genito-urinary region. If present in relatively small numbers, these organisms do little harm. If allowed to run rampant, however, they can cause many problems, with far-reaching consequences.

The most commonly-recognised form of the problem occurs in the vagina and is called thrush, or monillia, which has been recognised for hundreds of years. If you have this you will probably be aware of the symptoms which include itch or irritation, pain and sometimes swelling, accompanied by a white and usually smelly discharge. Once the mould has done its damage opportunistic bacteria can invade the area, setting up infections. This results in a change in the colour of the discharge from white to yellow.

Initially it was thought that the candidiasis when it occurred, was restricted to this area and could be dealt with by local vaginal treatment. The problem is that, once established in large numbers in the vagina, it is an

easy task for the *candida albicans* to migrate to the anus
and so travel up the digestive tract. Here it can cause
problems both locally and systemically as the toxins it
generates are absorbed into your bloodstream.

Conversely, if the increase in the number of the organisms starts in the intestinal tract and causes an initial
problem there, they can then migrate via the anus to the
vagina and cause local problems there.

The symptoms of systemic candidiasis include:

- Local problems within the digestive tract, such as
  wind, flatulence, alternating constipation and
  diarrhoea and an itchy anus. Because of the damage
  the mould does to the intestinal walls there is also
  diminished absorption of essential nutrients, which
  leads to general health problems associated with
  undernutrition. The damage also permits the
  absorption of partially-digested foods which can
  then set up allergic reactions.
- Nervous system symptoms include headaches, rapid
  mood swings from elation to depression, often
  without cause, irritability, anxiety, headaches and a
  feeling of being drunk or, as one patient put it,
  'woozy', poor memory and confusion and decreased
  motivation.
- A variety of food cravings can occur – cravings for
  sugar, alcohol, bread and other yeast-rich or pickled
  foods, plus cravings for the foods to which you have
  become allergic.
- Localised physical symptoms include sore throat and
  a coated tongue. Skin symptoms, cracks and flaking,
  commonly occur in folds or creases where there is
  moisture, such as between the buttocks, under the
  breast, between rolls of fat and between the toes
  (where it is commonly referred to as 'Athlete's Foot').
- You may also have pain in the muscles and joints

and you may have general allergic symptoms
including hayfever, asthma, sinusitis and more.

- PMS is a common symptom, as we shall see later in
this chapter, and anyone with this problem should
investigate the possibility that they have candidasis.
- You will probably feel tired, possibly even exhausted.
This can be caused both by the direct action of the
candida and by all the side effects that result from its
presence and activity.

The obvious question is why, since we all have *candida
albicans* in the digestive system, we don't all have these
symptoms. The answer lies in their number. You have
hundreds of different types and groups of organisms in
and on your body and the *candida albicans* group is only
one of these. If its numbers are kept in check by both
the type and quantity of the other organisms and by the
quality of the environment, and if your immune system
is healthy and keeps the *candida albicans* at bay, then you
can tolerate its presence and avoid the symptoms.

The trouble comes when *candida albicans* starts to take
over and become a significant part of your overall flora.
It then starts to cause symptoms. In time, when it
becomes a major inhabitant and when your immune
system has adjusted to it and no longer fights it
(particularly when you have not nourished and supported your immune system properly or have overloaded it with toxins), then a long-term situation
develops that is debilitating, often hard to diagnose and
difficult to alter.

There are many ways in which this explosion of *candida albicans* can happen. It can come about as the result
of a poor diet rich in sugar, refined carbohydrates and
alcohol plus an abundance of yeast-rich or fermented
foods which encourage *candida*. *Candida* also grows well
when you have below-normal output of stomach acid

and, as a result, secrete insufficient amounts of alkaline
digestive juices from the pancreas. The under-production
of stomach acid is, as we have already seen, a common
and often unrecognised problem. Your own immune
system *should* keep the *candida albicans* under control,
but when you have not given it all the nutrients it needs
and have overloaded it with other toxins, physical,
chemical and biological, *candida* has a chance to grow.
The use of antibiotics is a major cause of *candida* prolifer-
ation, both those you take when prescribed by your
doctor and those you get from food such as chicken and
from other intensively-reared animals, so is the use of
the contraceptive pill and of steroids such as cortisone.
The use of antibiotics and other drugs destroys many of
the beneficial organisms in your digestive tract, such as
lactobacillus acidophilus and *bifidobacteria*. These beneficial
organisms help the normal process of digestion, produce
vitamins that are beneficial to you and do not produce
toxins. Their loss leads to problems both as a result of
their absence and the presence of unwanted alternative
organisms such as *candida*. Stress in general both contributes to the problem and results from the problem in an
escalating spiral. Toxins and pollution can also add to
the problem of *candida* overgrowth.

Candida does damage in a number of ways:

- Firstly, just by existing in the digestive tract, it causes
  problems because of the toxins it produces and
  releases. One of these toxins is acetaldehyde which
  is also produced in the liver after you drink alcohol
  and contributes to the hangover feeling. This and
  other toxins that are produced lead to many of the
  symptoms associated with candidiasis.
- Secondly, *candida* is invasive and causes local damage
  to the mucosa such as the walls of the digestive
  tract. The areas where the intestinal walls are

damaged then allow partially-digested foods to cross
from the intestines into the bloodstream. Since this
partially-digested food is absorbed before it has
been completely broken down, it is recognised as a
foreign substance and your immune system tries to
protect you from it by attacking. As a result, you
become allergic to a variety of foods, usually the
ones you commonly eat and to which you are
exposed several times a day.

Avoiding the food is only a short-term solution.
The long-term answer is to deal with the *candida*
and heal your intestinal wall. Then, when you have
avoided your allergenic foods and repaired the
damage, you can usually reintroduce the foods with
safety. Until that time, the allergy symptoms that
result from this can cause many of the problems
related to fatigue and many of the problems that have
been listed above as being caused by *candida*.

Sometimes there are associated vaginal symptoms,
though not always. A possible scenario is as follows:

- You developed an infection of some sort, possibly
  far removed from either the vagina or the digestive
  tract.
- It was treated with antibiotics, which, while killing
  off the bacteria associated with the infection, also
  killed off the beneficial organisms in the digestive
  tract.
- This then allowed the *candida albicans* to proliferate
  in the digestive tract and spread to the vagina
  where it damaged the vaginal lining and led to a
  discharge, made up of mucous exudate, dead
  organisms and dead cells from the vaginal wall.
- It is a very simple step for the organisms to move
  from the anus to the vagina and vice versa so it can

easily spread back into the digestive system where its numbers support the *candida* already there as a result of oral antibiotics and the problem escalates.

• Meanwhile, back in the vagina, the damaged walls have created a wonderful environment for more bacteria and cystitis develops.

• More antibiotics are given to kill off the bacteria, this encourages the growth of more *candida albicans* and the problem worsens.

Notice that it is not the bacteria that cause the problem, rather, they take advantage of the tissue damaged by the *candida*, which in turn is encouraged by the use of antibiotics. Eventually, the *candida* has a strong hold, your symptoms become systemic, worsen and you are exhausted.

The problems this can cause can be devastating. Few women are interested in sex when they have vaginal thrush. Few are interested in sex when they are exhausted. Few are interested in sex when they have the emotional and mental symptoms described above. Neither the local symptoms nor the mental and emotional ones are conducive to a happy marriage and it is dismaying to think how many relationships, otherwise strong, may have foundered as a result of antibiotics, given possibly for a mild situation, such as a viral cold or flu, for which they don't even provide any benefit.

Candidiasis can be caused by the contraceptive pill. It can also occur in rhythm with a woman's menstrual cycle since progesterone, produced in the second half of the cycle, encourages its growth, and thus it can aggravate or even cause the symptoms labelled as PMS.

Since *candida* is present in everyone, in varying amounts, it is difficult to devise a test to indicate whether or not it is the culprit in your problem of fatigue. There are two common criteria that you can use. If you have

the symptoms listed above, then *candida* is a likely diagnosis. If you respond to the treatment programme it is
even more probable that it is what you had. Since the
symptoms are non-specific and since doctors only think
in terms of *candida* being a problem if there is obvious
vaginal thrush, or thrush in babies, it is possible you may
have had the problem, unrecognised, for many years. If
you see a practitioner who understands the problem,
they will want to take a thorough medical history and
to test both for yeast and mould sensitivities and for
allergies.

Patients with this problem frequently describe a long
history of having the symptoms, of many visits to doctors, of having a variety of tests done, all of which have
come back clear, and of being told there is nothing wrong
and it is 'all in their head', that they should 'pull themselves together and get on with things'. This worsens
the situation as not only do you feel bad and exhausted
but you start to doubt yourself too and to wonder if you
are indeed imagining things, yet at the same time
you also know that there is something wrong.

Cynthia is a typical example. She had three children, all
now at school. She had been tired, she told me, since
she'd married. She had put it down to the wedding, the
first child nine months later and the next two in the next
three years.

'But now', she said looking puzzled and slightly
ashamed, 'I should be feeling more energetic. There is so
much less to do with the children at school. We can even
afford help in the house now. Yet I keep feeling exhausted.
And I get so depressed. I'm happy one minute, then I
feel like bursting into tears. I used to put it down to
frustration, being cooped up in the house all day with
only the children to talk to, but now . . .' and her voice
trailed away in confusion. 'I've seen doctors, I've had

tests. They tell me there is nothing wrong, I should pull myself together and get on with my life. They're right, too, after all, I've got a life now that most women would envy. Sometimes, though, I think I'm going mad. Perhaps I am imagining things. Perhaps there really isn't anything wrong physically. Maybe I'm heading for a breakdown.' And with that she gave a short laugh that turned into a hiccup and then into tears, about which she was clearly both ashamed and embarrassed.

When I asked her to be specific it turned out that on their honeymoon she'd had a severe bout of cystitis, a new experience for her, which had been treated, unsuccessfully, with antibiotics. Only after they had come home and after several courses of treatment had the cystitis been eliminated, but the tiredness had started. She'd begun to experience digestive problems, bloating and flatulence, plus bouts of diarrhoea alternating with constipation, that she had attributed to the pregnancy rather than to developing candidiasis. After the birth, the symptoms had continued but been ignored or attributed to general fatigue, sleep disturbance and the emotional changes of motherhood. Further pregnancies, more antibiotics as the children became ill, and infections circulated, and by the time she saw me, she had a serious problem with systemic candidiasis. Vaginal thrush was only an occasional and mild problem and no one had pieced together the whole story.

Once she saw a complete picture that made sense to her, of when and how her problem had started and developed, she became much more positive. Instead of being told it was all in her head, she now had something positive and specific she could do. She participated fully in the entire treatment programme and recovered not only her health and energy but her happy disposition as well. Within a couple of months, her husband was commenting that she was once again, 'the girl he had

*married' and she was saying 'if only we'd known before,
I needn't have gone through this', and 'what if it hadn't
been recognised? I could have gone on feeling dreadful
for years'.*

The sad thing is that this is true. If candidiasis is not
recognised as the cause of the fatigue and all the other
symptoms, and the diagnosis *is* often missed, then
untold misery can result.

Exhaustion and fatigue typically occur at certain times
of life or in certain situations. Many of these are often
also times and situations where *candida* development is
most likely. In puberty, for instance, the changing hormone pattern leaves the body vulnerable to candidiasis.
Since this is accepted as a time when young people are
emotional or 'difficult', the symptoms due to *candida*
may be ignored. The tiredness may be put down to a
growth spurt, the stress of more serious exams, and the
emotional changes of dealing with approaching adulthood. This situation can be aggravated if teenage acne
develops and is treated with antibiotics. Tetracycline is
a particularly bad one to use.

The contraceptive pill increases the chance of candidiasis, yet here the emotional changes and other symptoms
may be blamed on the pill or the new relationship rather
than on the unsuspected *candida* problem.

Pregnancy is the time many women get thrush. The
local symptoms may be treated, but the emotional and
systemic symptoms and the tiredness may be attributed
to the pregnancy and the diagnosis of candidiasis may
be missed.

Men may well have skipped this chapter, thinking that
it does not apply to them. Yet men can get candidiasis.
It is less common, due in part to their different hormone
pattern and their different anatomy. Yet give a man antibiotics and he is nearly as likely to get intestinal thrush

as a women and may become tired as a result, along
with many of the other symptoms.

Candidiasis can cause exhaustion and is often a contributing factor even when other causes are involved.
When you are tired and run down you are much more
likely to develop candidiasis and it will aggravate existing exhaustion. You should certainly consider it as a
possible causative factor and check the situation out.

What To Do

The problem needs to be treated in two ways. It is clearly
important to treat the local area, be it vaginal thrush,
thrush in the throat or a skin problem. It is also essential
that you treat the digestive tract from where it causes
most of the system haevoc.

It is also true that a treatment programme that may
benefit one person will not work for another. Each individual is just that, an individual. Some people with candidiasis can eat vegetables, others react to many of them.
Some people with thrush can take vitamin C with
bioflavonoids, others react to the bioflavonoids and need
a synthetic vitamin C. Some people do well when biotin
is added to the therapy since it will reduce the conversion of the yeast form of *candida* to the mould form, but
others will feel worse since it can also increase the
growth rate of *candida*.

The following is a guide. However, there are so many
variables – such as whether you are infected with *candida*
or allergic to it (Chapter Twenty-four), whether your
possible bad symptoms following treatment are due to
die-off or a genuine bad reaction to the treatment, which
should be changed – that you may need the help of a
professional.

Local Treatment for Vaginal Thrush

- Douche with a mixture of about ten drops of propolis tincture in half a cup of aloe vera juice. This can be done night and morning. At night, after douching, apply and insert pure plain yoghurt (a spermicide dispenser tube is adequate).
- You can also make pessaries of an equal amount of pure propolis tincture and calendular tincture. Use sufficient gelatine to make the mixture set and apply while lying down.
- Apply aloe gel, using the applicator. It is soothing and healing.

Local Treatment for Thrush in the Digestive Tract

- Drink aloe vera juice – about a cup a day of a pleasant-tasting one. Provided it is still concentrated, this taste is a guide and suggests that all the bitter outer skin and spines have been removed. You don't want these as they can irritate the intestinal tract.
- Add ten drops of propolis tincture to the aloe vera juice and gargle with the mixture before you swallow it. This helps to dislodge the *candida albicans* from your mouth and throat. Propolis is made by bees and enables them to keep their hives free from moulds and bacteria.
- Another useful anti-fungal is garlic. Onion also helps though to a lesser extent, so eat plenty of these.
- Use olive oil as your oil of choice in salads and cooking since this can reduce the invasive ability of *candida*.
- Take a supplement containing hydrochloric acid if there is the slightest suggestion that you are producing insufficient stomach acid.
- Adding some of the good bacteria, the organisms that should be in the intestinal tract, helps to fight and

crowd out the *candida albicans*, so take *lactobacillus acidophilus* and *bifidobacteria*. If this is in powder form it should be kept refrigerated at all times and used up quickly. The alternative is to use a tablet form that is enterically coated, and some practitioners feel this is better than the powdered form. It too should be kept refrigerated.

- Roughage or fibre is important as it helps in the process of cleansing the intestines and absorbing and so removing the dead and unwanted organisms as well as preventing constipation and putrefaction.
- Improve your diet.

  Cut out sugar. This includes galactose, the sugar found in milk, glucose, fructose, sucrose as in 'sugar' and maltose from starch.

  Stop eating all foods containing yeasts or ferments including:
    – cheese, yoghurt and all soured and fermented dairy products, plus tofu
    – pizzas, buns, yeasted cakes, and all breads, even 'yeast-free', since there is still some activity there involving organisms or fermentation
    – smoked and cured meats, sausages such as salami and smoked fish
    – all alcohol except neat spirits (all alcohol would be even better)
    – soy and other sauces with a fermented or yeast base; Vegemite, Marmite, Bonox and other yeast spreads and drinks
    – mushrooms; all processed tomato products
    – dried fruits and fruits juices; all melons
    – vinegar, pickles, sauerkraut, mayonnaise (vinegar), olives
- Avoid junk foods and highly processed foods as they are commonly high in sugars, unwanted saturated fats and yeast-rich foods.

- If you are not a vegetarian, reduce your carbohydrate intake as far as possible and consume mainly protein foods and vegetables, at least until you are over the *candida* problem. The exception to this is if you have liver or kidney problem, in which case a high protein diet is not a good idea. If you are a vegetarian this is more difficult to achieve but at least make sure that your carbohydrates are complex and not refined.

Systemic Treatment

- Supplement with a full spectrum of vitamins and minerals, with particularly generous amounts of vitamin A and zinc to strengthen the mucosal wall, vitamin E for healing, vitamin C, some of the B vitamins and minerals such as zinc, manganese, copper and selenium to boost the immune system.
- Do not use antibiotics or the contraceptive pill, or take steroids.
- Eat free-range chicken and avoid meat from animals that may have been given antibiotics.

It is important, once you start the treatment, that you continue with it until it is complete and you are symptom-free. This can come about within days or weeks, or it may take months or longer. Much will depend on how long you have had it, how severe it is, how strictly you adhere to the above treatment guidelines and on your body's ability to recover. However long it takes, stick with it. There is some suggestion that if you stop the treatment part-way through you will have killed off the weaker *candida* organisms and left the stronger ones behind. If you stop at this point, it will be the strong ones that proliferate again and you will have a tougher opposition to fight next time.

Possible Side-Effect of Treatment – The Die-Off Effect

Many people report worsening of their symptoms when they start treatment for candidiasis. This comes about as a result of the effectiveness of the treatment. The treatment, if successful, causes the organisms to die, break open and release their toxins into the digestive tract. This will lead to a seeming aggravation of the problem. However provided you continue with the treatment, these symptoms will obviously be short-lived.

> *Sometimes when I warn a patient about the possibility of the die-off effect and its symptoms, it makes them anxious and disinclined to start the treatment. One woman refused point-blank. What was the point, she wanted to know, of starting a treatment that would cause her symptoms to worsen? She couldn't see beyond that to a resolution of her problem. After that, I took to making an oblique reference to it. I had told her that if any changes in her symptoms occurred before our next meeting she was to phone me. About five days later she did.*
>
> *'You said I should call, so I am. I feel dreadful, most peculiar, woozy. I have dreadful diarrhoea, lots of gas and I feel quite wiped out.'*
>
> *'Wonderful' was my response, and to her startled exclamation and query, I explained why. That was sufficient for her. Other patients get more concerned, so I call them into the practice and explain in more detail what is happening. I have found that as long as I am genuinely pleased at the changes, and not dismayed, they gain the confidence to understand what is happening and continue with the treatment.*

It is also possible that, as well as being infected by *candida albicans*, you had actually become allergic to it.

As with all allergens, there is the possibility of addiction and therefore of withdrawal effects. These withdrawal symptoms, as you cut yeasts out of your diet and eliminate the *candida albicans*, may, for a short while, seem even worse than the original problem.

If what you are doing is causing an increase in the symptoms, then you are probably on the right track. These symptoms should only last for a few days, or a week or two at most. If they continue, you will need to work with a practitioner who understands what is happening and can advise you.

References

Dr C.O. Truss, *The Missing Diagnosis*. 1982. Pub: C. Orian Truss MD

Dr W.G. Crook, *The Yeast Connection* 1983. Professional Books

See also:
Xandria Williams, 'Thrush: The Hidden Cause of Common Ailments'. *Australian Wellbeing*, Jan 1985 p.86.

Xandria Williams, *'Candida'. Prevention*, May 1989, p.95
(Copies available from the author.)

Chapter Seventeen

Bacteria, Viruses, Parasites and Other Organisms

In general, infections have the potential to pull you down and leave you feeling tired. Any infection and any organism is capable of doing this. However, if you are healthy, well-nourished and have an efficient and competent immune system, you are far less likely to succumb to infections than if your immune system is under-nourished and functioning inadequately. If your immune system is functioning relatively well but still succumbs the symptoms of the infection will be relatively mild and you will notice them far less than if the reverse was the case.

The same is true for the effect the organisms can have on your energy. If your immune system is relatively healthy, your adrenal glands are well nourished and you are getting all the nutrients you need, then an infection will lower your energy levels only slightly. If you are severely nutritionally compromised, your immune system has few reserves and you can succumb to the flu or pneumonia, a mild infection or repeated bouts of cystitis, a mild gastric upset or a severe reaction marked by debilitating diarrhoea and nausea, then in addition to all the other symptoms your energy levels will plummet.

It is inherent in the naturopathic view of health that

if you are fully fortified, nourished and one hundred per cent healthy, the bacteria and other organisms cannot get a hold. The organisms themselves do not initiate the health problem. However if they see the opportunity, if you are undernourished and ill-defended, they will move into your system and take hold.

If you get a mild viral cold you feel tired. If you get the flu, you feel more tired. If your sinuses become infected you feel even more tired and if you develop pneumonia, you become exhausted. The same is true if you get a kidney infection, a liver infection or a bronchial infection. Your digestive tract is also prey to infections. The common 'gastritis', which usually has more to do with the intestines than with the stomach, is a well-known experience after eating food that has 'gone off' and on which a variety of toxic bacteria have been living. Eating raw foods and drinking water in a variety of foreign countries is dangerous because of the organisms they can contain and to which you are unaccustomed, and the resulting symptoms, in addition to diarrhoea, usually include fatigue.

The smart answer to this type of fatigue is to give your immune system all the nutrients it needs to be fully healthy; then you will get the better of the infective agent. You may feel slightly tired while your body is fighting it but nothing like as tired as you will be if you succumb. Equally, it is worth reiterating that since many of these pathogens are around us all the time, you only tend to succumb if your body lets them in, if your ever-vigilant immune system lets them slip through the net or is unable to fight them. In other words, if you succumb to an infection, in the majority of cases the primary problem is not the pathogen but your inadequate immune system, and the exciting part about that notion is that this is something over which you can exert your authority and control.

The medical view and the view expressed here and
that of most natural or alternative therapists are dia-
metrically opposed. The medical approach is to give you
a drug, a foreign and usually toxic chemical, aimed at
killing the 'infectious' agent. The alternative view is that
you should boost your health so the agent can do you
no harm. This latter is actually a much easier thing to
do. You will never be able to kill off every single pathogen, so if you remain in an immune-compromised state
you will be forever vulnerable to any infectious agent
you meet. On the other hand, it is relatively easy and
much safer to rebuild your own immune system so you
can face all pathogens with a degree of complacency.

This does not mean that you take unnecessary risks.
No one, I hope, would be foolish enough to say that
because they are taking all the supplements their
immune system needs and are on a good diet, they need
not fear AIDS or take precautions. Even though their
risk is almost certainly a lot less than that of someone
whose immune system is less healthy it is foolish not to
take every precaution.

Viruses – They Are Not Alive

People often include viruses with bacteria and other
organisms, so a word of explanation is appropriate. Bacteria, parasites, moulds and other organisms are all
living creatures made up of cells – sometimes just one
cell, sometimes more. As such, they have a nucleus, like
a brain, that houses the genetic material, the DNA and
RNA. They also have organs (usually called organelles)
that are responsible for producing energy, eliminating
waste and reproducing substances they need. Further,
they can reproduce themselves, often by dividing in half.

Since they are alive they can also be killed. They can
be killed in a number of ways. They will die if their

energy production is interfered with, if they cannot process waste, if they cannot synthesise compounds they need, or if their metabolism is interfered with in some other way. Their numbers will diminish if they cannot reproduce. In other words they can be killed, just like you, by any agent that interferes with their normal life cycle.

For this reason, antibiotics can kill them. Antibiotics are substances that are *ant*agonistic to *bio*logical life. A variety of other substances and other organisms can also kill them.

Viruses are different. A virus is not made up of cells. It is not even a single cell. It is not a living thing. A virus is essentially a complex of genetic material and protein. Since it does not breathe, generate energy, eliminate waste, synthesise or reproduce, an agent (such as an antibiotic) that interferes with these processes has no effect on it.

You may argue that a virus does reproduce, that it grows in numbers and that a viral infection gets worse as the number of individual viruses increases. This is true, but does not mean they are alive and can reproduce themselves. Instead, a virus enters a living cell (as most molecules can do, this does not prove it's alive) and migrates to the nucleus of the cell (again, as certain molecules can do). Its DNA then effectively becomes the DNA or 'brains' of the cell. The cell is then instructed by this DNA to make more copies of the virus. The cell's reproductive machinery copies the virus until the cell becomes full of the virus. It then dies, breaks open, the viruses are spread around and are available for entry into other cells where the process is repeated. It's a bit as if a foreign intelligence took over your brain and instructed your body as to what it should do, eventually destroying it.

For this reason, there is absolutely no point in using

an antibiotic to treat a viral infection. Many doctors would argue that they give you an antibiotic when you get (viral) flu to ward off any bacteria that might be trying to invade as well. Yet we have already seen the damage that antibiotics can do (Chapter Sixteen) and so this rationale should be reassessed. The suggestion made here, of course, is that you should boost your own immune system so that bacteria are unable to get a hold.

Boosting your immune system also reduces the incidence of viral-induced infections and related health problems as it strengthens your cell walls so that they are capable of inhibiting the virus's entry. This suggestion, to improve your diet and lifestyle and take appropriate supplements, needs as many repeats as it takes finally to convince you to stop eating cakes and convert you to fruit instead, to stop you eating junk food snack meals and encourage you always to have fresh fruits and vegetables, etc. (and this means not just *some* fruit). For maximum results, it means *always* having fruit instead of cakes, biscuits and sweets, as well as taking your supplements *regularly*.

Haven't you ever wondered why some people are always getting colds, yet others, often working in the same office or living in the same house, don't. The latter are exposed to just the same bacteria and viruses as the former; it is simply that they have treated their body better than you have and their immune system is more effective. There is, of course, the question of genetics. Some people have to work harder to have a good immune system than do other people, but this is no reason to give up. It is a reason to take even more care of yourself.

Keep in mind that, since a virus isn't living and can't die, it can lodge in your tissues, usually within your immune system, lymph, spleen or liver, and stay there.

It may be there for years, totally inactive. Then when the situation is right, when you are run down or doing too much for the resources you have, it can get into a cell and start the infectious cycle already described. Once securely lodged in your system a virus can be there to stay. Your job is to keep the rest of you so healthy that the virus never gets a chance to break out. This is not (unwanted or inappropriate) suppression, it is (beneficial) containment. A bacterial infection might become more virulent if you suppress it but a virus, if contained, is inactive. On the other hand, it can become more virulent each time you let it take over and cause tissue damage.

In herpes, for instance, you may not get rid of the virus or dislodge it totally from your system once it has entered. What you can do is prevent it surfacing. Again, this is not a case of disadvantageous suppression of the problem, since 'letting it out' in no way implies that you will get rid of it, merely that it will be active for a while and then settle down into a back seat again, at least for a while. Keep in mind that this is a case of containment, of preventing it expressing itself and creating the well-known symptoms.

Viruses and Fatigue

There are two main viruses that have been associated with CFS, assuming you already have an immune system that was vulnerable enough to let them in in the first place. Both of them are related to the herpes, shingles and chicken pox viruses. They are Cytomegalovirus (CMV) and the Epstein-Barr Virus (EBV), the virus involved in many cases of infectious mononucleosis or glandular fever.

If you succumb to EBV, you may never get rid of it. It may always be lodged somewhere in your system.

Provided you maintain a healthy immune system this may cause you little or no problem. If you succumb to some other infection, become stressed or overtired, get candidasis or some other load is placed on you, the EB virus may get its chance, make a break and cause you to become exhausted.

Stress is such an easy concept to ignore, yet when you are stressed your body produces a variety of compounds, some of which can make it a lot easier for the virus to surface. This is one of the reasons you are advised to change the way you react to situations. Remember: it is not the situation that is stressful, it is the way you react to it – otherwise everyone would be stressed by the same situations and clearly this is not the case. So find ways to reduce the things in your life that you find stressful and to change your responses as well. In this way you can assist your body in defending itself against viruses.

A variety of chemical substances can also cause a virus to proliferate. It appears that many of the chemical toxins in our environment can do this. Even some plants, beneficial in many circumstances, can do this, including some of the anti-inflammatory herbs such as echinacea, feverfew and devil's claw. Other substances can do the same thing, including some varnishes, paints, building materials and clothing materials that contain Tung Oil.[1]

Vitamin C Treatment

One of the best ways of helping your body defend itself against CMV, EBV and other viruses is to take massive doses of vitamin C in a carefully planned way. Drs Linus Pauling, Robert Cathcart and Irwin Stone and others have used and promoted this for decades. If you are taking vitamin C orally, here is what you should do when you want to fight a viral outbreak.

Oral vitamin C

Using either the sodium ascorbate or ascorbic acid form of vitamin C as a powder (*not* calcium ascorbate):

- take 1 teaspoon every half hour until you experience flatulence and the beginning of diarrhoea.
- then reduce the dose, the frequency or both so that you continue to experience flatulence but *just* avoid the diarrhoea.

Your aim is to take as much vitamin C as you can absorb. Once you get diarrhoea, you are consuming more than you can absorb. If you slow down to a point where you no longer have digestive symptoms, you are not consuming as much as you could absorb. You need to get your body as near to saturation as you can. Contrary to medical fears, there is no proven case to suggest that you increase your risk of getting kidney stones when you do this and there is even some evidence to the contrary, that you may actually reduce the risk. As you start to beat the virus, you will find you can take less and less vitamin C before you reach your threshold.

If the treatment has been completed successfully you should find in future that by taking only a few teaspoons a day you quickly reach saturation, indicated by slight flatulence. You should also find that many of your symptoms have gone and you feel more energetic. If not, then repeat the full treatment again. If this is still not sufficient, particularly when combined with all the other suggestions in this book for improving your overall health in general and the state of your immune system in particular, you may need to get intravenous vitamin C (see below).

This process works for all viruses, from those that cause the common cold to those that cause EBV and

CMV. There is also evidence that it has helped people suffering from the AIDS virus [R. Cathcart pers. comm.].

> *I recall a patient who had had glandular fever a couple of years previously and was still suffering from the effects. When I saw him, he was at last back at work, in a stressful job in the television industry. However, it took him all his time and energy to get to work, do his job and go home and sleep, preferably for at least twelve hours a night. At the weekend he did little else but sleep and rest. After a week on this high vitamin C regime, plus a general supplement programme, he was up to socialising again and had taken on a new lease of life.*

Intravenous vitamin C

It may be that you cannot take in sufficient vitamin C by mouth and may need to get it intravenously. When this happens, the change in the symptoms and the increase in energy can seem almost miraculous. You will need to find a practitioner who gives IV vitamin C and discuss the amount required. You should continue to take as much as you can by mouth and use the IV vitamin C to 'top up' until you have sufficient to overcome the problem.

This vitamin C treatment is important if you are tired or get frequent infections. It is almost essential if you have CFS.

Parasites

Parasitic infections are among the most widespread diseases we have. They can cause a variety of direct symptoms. They can also reduce or suppress the normal immune response and thus cause other problems to occur and we have already seen that a poor immune system can lead to a number of health problems that in turn contribute to fatigue.

If you suspect a parasitic infection you would be well advised to have this checked out and to take the appropriate action, depending on the parasite, to eliminate it. This area is too extensive to cover here, but your therapist should be able to help you.

Other Organisms

Just as almost any health problem causes fatigue, so any organism may adversely affect your health. One that has cropped up several times among my patients is giardia. This is commonly thought of as a tropical problem affecting the digestive tract, but it does also occur in cooler climates (aggravated, perhaps, by the growing ease and frequency of international travel). I have had several patients who have had giardia, traced its origin back to a probable source and realised that their fatigue started around the same time. This is not the place to go into the full symptoms and treatments of parasitic, bacterial and other pathogens. However, if you have recently travelled and have experienced symptoms you associate with your trip, or if you have any symptoms about which you are concerned, get professional advice and ask about the possibility of pathogens being present.

What Your Immune System Needs

Your immune system is a part of your body and needs all the nutrients that you do. Go back to the chapters on nutrition in general (Three to Seven) and treat your body and your immune system with the consideration they need and deserve. You will also find reference to the nutrients your immune system needs in Part IV.

Again, if you think you have read and heard all this

before, are you doing enough about it? Probably not. It is all too easy to say 'just one piece of cake, just one biscuit, just one packet of fatty and salty chips . . . won't matter.' It will. Each time you eat such a food you are not only loading up on the toxins, sugars and fats, but you are also going without more nutritious food. It is often just as easy to say 'Well, everyone eats like this, so why shouldn't I?' The answer is that either they too are sick (though you may not be aware of it), or they have a more resilient genetic make-up than you. Either way, if you want to be healthy and have lots of energy, take the proper care of yourself. It is up to you, and no one else, to see that you produce all the energy of which you are genetically capable, unimpeded by unwanted viruses, bacteria, parasite and other organisms.

References

[1] Brighthope, I, *Fighting fatigue, and the Chronic Fatigue Syndrome.* McCulloch Publishing 1990, Allen and Unwin, 1991.

Chapter Eighteen

Allergies and Sensitivities

The term 'allergies' can mean different things to different people and we are going to give brief consideration to several aspects and types of allergies here.

Firstly there is the distinction between the classical or conventional 'allergy' and the broader concept of allergies as used by many clinical ecologists and natural therapists. Conventional allergies are considered to be a person's idiosyncratic reaction to a substance, plant or organism, a reaction that most other people do not experience but that results from certain specific changes within the body of the sufferer including the production and presence of antibodies and the release of histamine.

This allergic reaction cannot occur on the first exposure to the substance as there are no antibodies to the substance pre-existing within your body. These antibodies can, however, develop as a result of the first exposure and you can react either on the second or some subsequent exposure. This subsequent exposure could be the next day or years later, regardless of any exposures in between. Since histamine is often released by the allergic response in this type of allergy, antihistamines are commonly used in the treatment.

Allergies differ from toxins in a number of ways. A substance that is a toxin will generate symptoms in anyone exposed to it. In addition, a toxin will produce symptoms on the first exposure and there is no need for the presence of pre-existing antibodies. Further, toxins will produce a similar symptom pattern in everyone. On the other hand, only allergic people react to substances with allergic symptoms and a substance that is an allergen to one person may not be an allergen to another person. Further, allergens can produce quite different symptoms in different people. For instance some people may react by developing skin conditions such as hives or eczema whereas others could react by developing respiratory symptoms such as sinusitis, hay fever or asthma.

Secondly, in addition to this strict definition, there is a broader concept of allergies. According to this definition, you are considered to be allergic (or sensitive) to a substance if it causes idiosyncratic reactions, whether or not you have specific antibodies against the substance or histamine is released. These symptoms are commonly 'masked' rather than immediate and obvious, and it is usually impossible to tell what you react to by simple observation.

The symptoms will vary from person to person. They could include (but are not restricted to) mental symptoms, including a huge variety of mood changes and altered levels of alertness, memory and ability to concentrate, plus energy disturbances from mild lethargy to severe exhaustion. Other symptoms may involve the respiratory system, from sinus problems and hay fever to asthma; the cardiovascular system, particularly rapid or erratic heart rate; the skin, from a mild itch to total body dermatitis and eczema; a variety of digestive upsets, including gas, flatulence and diarrhoea; joint problems from swelling and oedema to destructive arthritis; kidney problems and many more.

Our concern here focuses on the fatigue and exhaustion. This may be a specific and immediate primary symptom that results from exposure to the substances concerned. The loss of energy can also be a secondary effect, aggravated and prolonged by the effect of the allergens (the substances causing the allergic response) on the rest of the body – the heart and the lungs, for instance.

So far, we have considered substances that are a normal, natural and usually safe part of our environment – foods, plants, insects and so forth. Most people have no problem with them, a few are allergic or sensitive to them and should avoid them.

The third part of the problem comes about when we consider sensitivities in general in relation to all the toxic chemicals in the environment (see Chapter Eight). Here we are dealing with substances that are toxic to everyone, to a greater or lesser extent. These toxic reactions are often known and listed. But when considering allergies, we have to consider the people who have become acutely sensitive to some of these substances, in addition to their usual toxic effects. These above-and-beyond reactions of the sensitive individual are sometimes considered, at least by the person suffering from them, to be allergic reactions; they can also be called acute sensitivities that add to the fundamental toxic reaction. An obvious example is the person who not only has candidiasis but, in addition, has developed an allergic reaction to *candida albicans*.

This is not the place to go into a full discussion of allergies or how to deal with them. The books by Randolph[1] are classics in this area, and there are others that can assist you in the daily and practical methods of dealing with allergens.[2] Our purpose here is to point out how allergies could be affecting your energy level. However, a few points are pertinent to help you understand the situation and the following are some of the most commonly-asked questions about allergies and sensitivities.

Q. Why do I react when other people don't?
A. Each person is an individual. Roger Williams coined the concept of 'biochemical individuality' several decades ago. He recognised that, while people looked relatively similar on the outside, internally there are much greater differences physically and huge differences chemically. For instance, most people fall within a height range of five foot to six foot four, a variation of plus or minus about twelve per cent about the mean. Internally, one person's stomach can be twice the size of another person's, possibly even more, a variation of over thirty per cent or more about the mean. Chemically, one person's need for a nutrient can be several times that of another person's, a variation of several hundred per cent.

Similarly, people are unique in the way they respond to a variety of substances including those found in foods and the chemicals added to the environment. Most people can drink milk, some can drink large amounts. Others can drink a small amount but react to the lactose (milk sugar) if they drink more. A few allergic individuals are highly reactive, whether the amount is large or small, and may show a variety of symptoms, including fatigue, following the consumption of even a few drops.

I recall a patient who was suffering from schizophrenia. His mother was doing a fantastic job, giving him all the supplements he needed and obtaining a gradual, though mild, improvement. We did allergy tests on him and found he was allergic to milk. She had been giving him his tablets crushed and mixed into a thick chocolate milkshake. When she stopped doing this and cut all dairy products out of his diet he became much calmer and more rational. All was well as long as milk was kept out of his diet, but since he loved it, this was difficult. After finding and drinking a carton of it, he became exceedingly violent. Sadly, he was then put into a home where they refused to recognise his milk allergy and allowed him as much as he wanted.

As another example, everyone will experience some reaction to the toxic effects of carbon tetrachloride; others will show an acute and much greater reaction and may get severe symptoms after the smallest exposure. To add a further dimension to 'biochemical individuality', each person may react with a different group of symptoms, even if the causative allergenic agent is the same.

Q. Why am I reacting now, when I have been exposed to that food/plant/creature/substance all my life with no problems until recently?
A. It's a bit like stressing a piece of steel. Initially you may be able to bend it this way and that without it weakening, then a 'breaking point' occurs and it develops a 'crease' such that next time it is stressed it immediately gives way along this stress line. In the same way, it is possible that initially your body coped with exposure to the substance. With repeated exposures, it is weakened and, once weakened, even a small exposure will cause major problems and symptoms. A new pattern has been set.

Edwina was thirty-five when she came to see me because of arthritis.

'I am much too young,' she insisted, 'to have arthritis. Even mother doesn't have it yet, though grandmother does.'

Based on a symptoms group that suggested allergies (she had eczema and occasional bouts of hay fever), we did the tests and found her to be allergic to peanuts, turkey and tomatoes.

I explained that a reaction to tomatoes was common when arthritis occurred, but it was the turkey and peanuts that really upset her. She was a flight attendant and used to snack on the packets of peanuts not wanted by passengers and turkey was her favourite meat.

'Why those?' she queried. 'I love them, I've eaten them for years, for the past six years anyway, since I've been flying. They didn't cause problems before.'

Maybe they didn't, but the arthritis in her hip certainly disappeared when she gave them up. I also suggested to her that they may have been doing damage for a while but that it had taken this long to show up as arthritic damage of sufficient severity to cause pain.

Your digestive system and your immune and defence systems have to be considered. They may have protected you for years, but now, after years of a diet that has probably been nutritionally inadequate and years of exposure to a variety of other stressors, other health risks, infections, toxins and so forth, added to the possible decrease in your production of stomach acid and digestive enzymes, the total load has become too much. You were living on capital, and at some point the capital ran out.

This can happen even when there is only the normal or low level of exposure. It can also happen after a major overload. Perhaps you only drank a small amount of milk in your tea, then you went on a milk and banana weight-loss diet and drank two or three glasses of milk a day. This high exposure may have been enough to tip you over into an induced allergic reaction to milk that has remained with you ever since, and you are now reactive even when you only have a teaspoon of it in your tea.

Or take the case of one patient of mine. Recently widowed, she had sold the family home, bought a flat, moved in and painted it throughout. Exposure to the paint fumes twenty-four hours a day had induced a chemical sensitivity to the paint such that she eventually had no choice but to sell it and move into another flat. Even the small quantity of chemicals degassing from the dry paint, months later, had become sufficient to cause her symptoms of headaches, confusion, anxiety, tiredness and more.

Further, the gradual accumulation of repeated exposures to a substance to which you have become sensitive can gradually damage organs and interfere with the functioning of different parts of the body. The first you may know of this is when this progressive damage reaches a point where overt symptoms occur. The substance was causing you problems all along, but they were below your threshold of awareness. Arthritis is a good example of this. You may have been reacting allergically to several foods for years and they may have been acting on your joints, initially with only minimal damage and no obvious symptoms. In time, the effect has accumulated, symptoms have started, you have become aware of them and are now wondering why you have 'suddenly' become allergic.

Once this happens, there is an additional danger. Since your system is overloaded you can now easily and rapidly become allergic to a variety of new substances, even substances which you could previously consume with ease and which now 'suddenly' disagree with you.

Q. If I am allergic or sensitive to a substance, why do I not react every time I am exposed to it?
A. You may react only when you are tired, or only when your diet has been worse than usual and your intake of

nutrients has been down. You may react only when you
have been exposed to a variety of other allergens at the
same time, or only to a specific combination of certain
allergens. The total complex of the chemical and allergen
load, plus the state of your body's health, nutrition and
immune function at a specific time, have to be considered.

One day you may (just) be able to cope with all the
chemicals at work, go home thrilled with the energy you
have and decide to use it to clean the oven (sprays), do
the ironing (more sprays to make the job easy), celebrate
with a well-earned glass of wine (yeasts) and then sit in
front of television (electromagnetic field). This may be a
definite overload but the symptoms may not show until
you are in the office next morning. This time you *do*
feel bad at work and blame the office air-conditioning.
Feeling tired that evening, you do little but prepare a
balanced meal, which you digest easily while you relax
over a good book and take your supplements. Next day
you *can* cope with all the toxins the office can throw
at you until the end of the day, so now you think maybe
the office environment isn't the problem after all. However, when you get home and have a glass of wine, that
is the last straw – you start to feel exhausted and this
continues the next day as you arrive at work. By then
you are confused. What do you do? Do you blame the
exhaustion during the second morning on the office
chemicals of the day before, or on what you did in
the evening? Possibly the latter. Yet you should actually
blame both: the variation in symptoms is simply evidence of the total load to which you were exposed and
the way your body handled it.

One way to resolve this situation is to be aware of
how you feel during the weekend. This will often help
you to distinguish between office- or work-related toxins
and allergens and those that occur outside the work-

place. Yet again, there may be a specific combination of reactions that occur only at weekends – say, the combination of deeply-inhaled pollutants as you play tennis by a main road plus the effect of yeasts as you drink additional, social quantities of alcohol. You may not blame the alcohol since you also drink during the week, not recognising that the pollutants were the last straw that meant you could no longer handle the alcohol (yeasts).

If all this sounds confusing, it is. You may be able to sort it out for yourself, but it is more likely that you will need the help of someone who understands allergies, clinical ecology and toxic reactions in their various combinations.

Q. Why do tests show I am allergic to a food, yet I can eat it and not get any obvious symptoms?
A. Many, if not most, allergy reactions are 'masked'. This means that the body has, in effect, adapted to the allergen and has learnt to deal with the symptoms in a chronic and more prolonged way. There is no acute reaction, no sudden flare-up of hives, for instance, immediately after you consume or are exposed to the offending substance. Instead, there is a steady effect on the brain, perhaps causing confusion and the feeling of living in a fog, or an effect on the adrenal glands, reducing your ability to create energy when you need it. All the other symptoms you experience may be a gradual accumulation of the ongoing effect of the allergens rather than a specific acute response to a single exposure.

It's a bit like floodwaters. Protective catchment dams can be built. This means that instead of episodic and sudden rushes of water, there will be a steady flow, causing minor flooding all the time instead of major destruction less frequently. The storage dam can smooth the effect out, but the long-term damage is still being done.

Q. I have already had my allergies tested. I avoided the foods for a while but then I found I had major reactions even when I ate only a small amount. I was worse off than before. It doesn't make sense, what should I do?

A. This is very clearly explained by Rinkel, Randolph and Zeller (1951) who described nine stages when dealing with allergies.[1]

In Stage 1 (Food Sensitivity) you experience your normal, masked and unrecognised reaction to the allergenic foods. In Stage 2 (Unmasking) you avoided the food for up to four days. Stage 3 (Hyperacute Clinical Reaction) lasts for eight days or more. If you are exposed to the food during this time, you experience acute symptoms. These can be either severe and disturbing, or mild but definitely noticeable. Stage 4 (Active Sensitisation with Omission) covers the time during which you continue to avoid your allergens and your degree of sensitivity gradually decreases.

The next stage is Stage 5 (Latent Sensitisation with Omission), during which time you can consume the substance once and experience no reaction yet get a reaction after repeated exposures. This comes about because the first exposure reactivates your allergic response. This stage is usually confusing to people because they conclude that since the food didn't cause symptoms the first time, the reactions experienced after the second exposure cannot have been due to it but must have been caused by something else. Stage 6 (Tolerance) means you have finally arrived at a level of safety. There is some suggestion that complete tolerance is never achieved and that, if you eat the offending food often enough and in sufficient quantity you may become allergic to it again. This tolerance has come about via a lot of self-discipline and careful eating; it would be a pity to lose it by repeated high exposure.

In Stage 7 (Tolerance after Addition of Food), you can eat some of the allergic foods again without losing what you have so laboriously gained. Provided you have eaten the food only occasionally, you will remain tolerant and without symptoms, either overt or covert. How much food can be tolerated before tolerance is lost is individual and may, at the practical level, be difficult to determine, so avoidance except where this would be socially diffi-cult is recommended. Do not, for instance, decide to have pizzas three nights a week if you are allergic to yeast, cheese, tomato paste, mushrooms and anchov-ies – a common occurrence if you have candidiasis or are sensitive to moulds and yeasts. On the other hand, if there are some breadcrumbs on your veal or fish, if there is some tomato purée in the casserole or a sprink-ling of cheese on the salad, you probably need not be concerned, provided you really have reached Stage 7.

A worthwhile practice, if you want to be sure you are not re-sensitising yourself to the foods to which you were allergic, is to have at least four days between each exposure to these foods. If you are exposed too often, you move on to the next stage.

In Stage 8 (Latent Sensitisation with Usage of Food) you are on the slippery slope back into allergic sensi-tivity. Your body is returning to a state whereby reactions to the food or substance are occurring with increasing frequency. The longer you remain in this stage, the longer it will take you to become tolerant again should you return to avoidance and cease to be exposed. Stage 9 (Acute Sensitisation with Usage of Food) is accompanied by the recurrence of acute reactions each time you eat the food and leads back to Stage 1 (Masked Food Sensitisation).

All this may seem somewhat contrived to you, but it does provide a useful basis for understanding the changes that occur and helps to answer the questions posed above. The Stages are not always clear-cut and are often difficult to define, yet the overall concept can help you to understand your reaction to allergenic foods in different circumstances before, during and after avoidance.

Q. Why do I crave some of the things to which I am allergic. Why do they seem to make me feel good?
A. There are many different reasons for this. Some allergens or sensitivities act on specific receptor sites in the brain. These are often, but not exclusively, the grains and dairy products if you are allergic to them. The receptor sites are like the opiate receptors on which morphine and other drugs act, including the body's own natural painkillers. Part of this reaction is to make you feel good initially, creating the addiction. When the sensation wears off there is a counter-reaction and you feel bad or let down. Not surprisingly, you recognise that the substance made you feel good and in an effort to recapture that feeling, you choose (crave) the food. I have had grown men cry when told they could no longer consume milk (their addictive allergy) in any form, and patients choose not to return when they knew I expected them to give up certain foods (to which they were addicted). As one woman said, many years ago, 'I'm going to find another practitioner, one who doesn't say I have to give up bread.'

Some allergens react by sending your blood sugar levels up. This gives you a burst of energy and you feel great. Then, as the insulin is released and does its job of directing this glucose out of the bloodstream and into the cells (see Chapter Fifteen), your blood sugar level falls. If other hormones do not act to keep it up, your low blood sugar level can leave you feeling dreadful. Understandably, you want the good feeling back and so consume more of the reactive food.

People rarely associate these later and unpleasant reactions with the allergen. They do associate the initial, pleasurable, reaction with them so they go back for more, thus setting the cycle off yet again. It is not possible to specify the allergens that will do this since the effect is more a function of the way your body responds to allergens than of the specific allergen.

Q. Why am I suddenly getting a lot of new allergies? It seems that every time I eat something new it is all right for a while and then I start reacting to it. I was better off before I changed my diet or did anything.
A. Not so, but this is where some professional advice may be needed. Once you have stressed both your immune system and your detox processes to the limit and they are working to capacity, you have no reserves left. When this is combined with diminished output of stomach acid and digestive enzymes plus the presence of inappropriate organisms in your digestive tract, all of which lead to diminished digestive capacity, the problem escalates. Your body is then particularly susceptible to any new toxins. It is susceptible to the absorption of any partially digested food, even to substances that it handled before, and it is all too easy for new allergens to develop When the dam floods, everything is carried over and new sensitivities are created.

To help prevent the creation of new allergies, it is important to keep your diet as varied as possible. You may laugh at this, having just been given a list of all the foods you must avoid, probably foods that make up a large proportion of your diet, and feeling that you have less food choices than before, not more, yet the need is there. Most people's diet is comprised of relatively few

foods and many other choices are available. You probably eat some fruits and some vegetables yet find, when
you check out the full list of all that is available in the
shops, that there are many other types you could eat.
You probably eat mainly wheat and possibly some oats
or rye, yet there are many other grains and flours you
could eat, including millet, rice, buckwheat (not a grain
strictly speaking, but it does substitute for grains); or
you could use sago and tapioca either whole or ground
into a flour, and there are flours made from legumes
such as soy, chick peas and lentils. You probably eat
peanuts and rarely consider all the other nuts available.
There are almost certainly dozens of different foods that
you could be eating.

The reason why this variety is important is that if you
already have allergies you have shown that you have a
tendency to develop them. This being the case, if you
change from eating wheat daily to eating barley daily,
you could well develop an allergy to barley, whereas
if you have a much wider variety of foods with less
frequent exposure you are less likely to develop new
allergies.

The answer to this scenario is not to focus all your
attention on avoiding everything that causes you problems. The answer is, certainly, to reduce your load of
toxins and avoid your allergens, but to further assist the
process by doing all you can to improve your nutrition
and repair your immune system. In this way, you can
boost your ability to handle the existing toxins *and* repair
any organs or tissues that have been damaged. Stand and
rebuild, rather than flee from all allergens and toxins, is
obviously sensible advice, but this should, at least
initially, be combined with avoidance.

If your problem is not general fatigue and lack of
energy combined with allergies, but has progressed and
become full CFS, the instructions will almost certainly

be a lot more strict. You should then avoid all your allergens entirely, paying particular attention to the nine-stage sequence described above. You should avoid all toxins, even going to considerable and often inconvenient lengths to do so.

Detecting Allergies

This is not the place to go into a more detailed discussion of allergies, to establish whether or not you do have allergies and to explore all the possible ways of detecting them. That is a specialised job. There are books that cover these topics and you will probably derive even greater benefit from consulting a professional. There are also books that explain in detail how to handle the situation once you have established your allergies, how to avoid them, substitutes to use, tricks to be wary of when reading food labels and so forth (Williams, 1987).

We have already alluded to the fact that testing for food allergies using skin pricks is not the best way. In fact those results are, according to Randolph and others, more often wrong than right. The ultimate testing involves total abstinence from a food for four days and then a challenge with sublingual drops. However, this method is both too specialised and much too dangerous for an individual to try on their own. It is also extremely time-consuming.

There are other tests that are nearly as accurate and useful and that are easier to administer.

- The cytotoxic test involves a trained specialist taking 5 ml of your blood and then mixing a drop of your blood with a drop of each specially-prepared food solution and observing whether or not the white cells die.
- The pulse test involves measuring your pulse before

eating a food, then eating the food and measuring your pulse immediately afterwards and at fifteen-minute intervals. If it rises by more than ten per cent it could be that you are allergic to the food. Clearly this method will only show allergens if one of their symptoms is to stimulate the heart to beat faster.

- Applied kinesiology, or muscle testing, involves measuring the resistance of your arm, held out sideways and horizontally, to downward pressure on your hand either before and after eating the food or, more usually, before and after putting some of the food on your tongue. If you spit it out afterwards, rather than swallowing it, you can test several foods one after the other in this way.

Of these, I have found the cytotoxic test to give the most useful results, but the other two methods can also be helpful and have the advantage of being ones with which you can experiment for yourself.

Allergies Are Often Missed

Finally, it is worth suggesting that allergies are often overlooked or missed as a diagnosis. If you have done all you can to improve your energy, even if you have no obvious symptoms of allergies, it is worth testing for them on the chance you have masked food allergies. If you do have allergies and do not detect them, trying to improve your health and increase your energy is like trying to play cat's cradle with only one hand.

References

[1]Randolph, T.G., and Moss. R.W., *An Alternative Approach to Allergies*. Lippincott and Crowell, 1979

Rinkel, H.J. Randolph, T.G. and Zeller, M., *Food Allergy*. Charles C Thomas, 1951
(Both classic books on the subject.)

[2]Williams Xandria, *Living with Allergies*, Allen and Unwin, 1987.

Chapter Nineteen

Cardiovascular Problems

There are many potential problems related to your heart and circulation system that could be heralded by the onset of fatigue. We have already discussed the anaemias. It is time now to consider some of the other problems that relate to the heart and of which fatigue could be one of the first early warning signs.

Heart Problems

Almost everyone with a heart problem of any sort will complain of feeling tired. Lack of energy may not necessarily be the major symptom but it is a very common one and may well, at the start, even be the only one. At the time it may not be recognised as the first symptom heralding a heart problem, but it is common to find, when the history is reviewed, that there was a period of unusual and increasing fatigue before the onset of more specific symptoms such as angina or palpitations.

Your heart is essential, not only for life, but for the production of energy. Your heart is an intimate and essential part of the flow of blood throughout the body and it is the blood that carries the oxygen needed by all the cells for the conversion of food into energy. Without an adequate supply of oxygen, you cannot produce an adequate amount of energy. In other words, if there is insufficient output of fresh, oxygenated, blood from the heart, all the other tissues will suffer from lack of oxygen and thus will have reduced capacity to burn or oxidise the three major fuels, carbohydrates, fats and proteins, and produce energy.

Although the incidence of death from cardiovascular diseases is declining somewhat in Western societies, it is still the major killer, accounting for approximately fifty per cent of deaths. Thus, since one of the symptoms of cardiovascular inadequacy is fatigue, it is important that the possibility of a heart problem is either ruled out or attended to.

Nutrients for the Heart

The heart is one of the busiest organs in your body. It beats from birth to death without ever taking a rest. It is therefore no surprise to find that it needs so many nutrients. There are several nutrients particularly important for the heart. Your nutrient intake is something over which you can exercise control and by knowing what nutrients your heart needs in particular you can go a fair way to preventing our number one killer.

Magnesium and potassium are two important minerals. They work with the nervous system and help the heart to maintain its normal rhythm.

There has to be a proper balance of sodium and potassium in the body, yet with the common and excessive addition of salt to the diet, in food processing, during cooking and at the table, you are likely to have an excess of sodium and a relative deficiency of potassium. This is aggravated by the increased urinary loss of potassium when diuretic drinks such as tea, coffee and alcohol are drunk and when diuretic medications are used. When medical diuretics are prescribed, Slow-K (a potassium supplement) is sometimes, though not always, prescribed. However, no allowance is made for the other minerals lost by increased urination and the loss of magnesium induced by the diuretics can have an adverse effect on your heart.

Derick Watson came to see me initially because he was getting cramps in his legs. He was sixty-three, with high blood pressure and high cholesterol. He was still relatively fit, playing a gentle game of tennis at the weekend. As we talked, however, he admitted to a general fatigue and to the thought that he'd soon have to give up his tennis. But the real problem at the moment was that he was sleeping poorly, a fact he put down to the cramps he got during the night and a feeling, as he put it, of restlessness in his legs. He was on diuretic medication for his high blood pressure and was taking Slow-K.

I suggested he took a combined calcium (500 mg) and magnesium (500 mg) supplement, which stopped the cramps and gave him more relaxed sleep (calcium will do this mentally as well as physically); vitamin E, starting with 50 mg a day and building up to 500 mg a day (with checks on his blood pressure as this can rise, in a few people, if you go to a high dose immediately), which stopped the restlessness; and a general multivitamin complex with 50 mg of most of the B vitamins for his overall health and energy. Within a few weeks, he reported feeling a lot better overall and no inclination to give up his tennis.

Another common mineral pair is calcium and magnesium. This pair should also be in a proper balance. Most people are aware of the need for calcium. It is needed for bones, teeth and nails and to prevent osteoporosis. It is the most common reason people feel that milk is so important in their diet and many people take supplements of it to protect their bones. However, magnesium is just as important yet is rarely taken as a supplement, this is unfortunate since the average Western diet is deficient in magnesium. The Ten-State survey done some years ago in the US showed that 70% of people consumed less than the RDA of magnesium. Another study showed that the magnesium content of the soil had dropped by 50% between 1953 and 1973 and there is little to suggest that there has been a reversal in this pattern. On top of this, only 10% of Americans consume the recommended amount of vegetables, a major source of magnesium.

People prone to magnesium deficiency are the young and the elderly, people who drink alcohol, people under stress or with health problems and people on drug medications. A lack of magnesium in an otherwise adequate diet fed to experimental animals has been shown to lead to damage to the heart and the arteries, damage that can be cured by adding magnesium back into the diet.[1]

The amino acid, aspartic acid, is preferentially taken up by the heart muscle. Thus, when bound to aspartic acid, both potassium and magnesium can be specifically targeted to the heart in preference to other tissues in the body. Thus K-Mag, or potassium magnesium aspartate, is a mineral and amino acid supplement often recommended for people suffering from heart problems, particularly those related to the rhythm of the heart beat.

Taurine is another amino acid needed by the heart, although not one that is incorporated into proteins. Its main functions are in the liver, where it is involved in the formation of bile. In the heart, it helps to maintain the potassium balance.

Carnitine is also an amino acid that is not a part of protein. It is made in the body in a process which involves two other amino acids, methionine and lysine, and vitamin B6, as we have seen (Chapter Five). Although not used in protein building, it, like taurine, has specific metabolic roles in the body. One of these is to facilitate the process of converting fats into energy in the muscles. To achieve this, the fats that are in the bloodstream have to enter the cells where they are partially broken down; the fragments then have to enter the mitochondria, the sub-units within the cells where the major part of combustion of the fats and carbohydrates takes place. Carnitine facilitates this process and without it, it is possible to have starving cells being bathed in a sea of fats yet unable to benefit from them. This is also a reason why you can eat and yet have no energy.

Without carnitine, you cannot utilise the fuels in the food you eat, so you still feel tired and continue to eat, thus gaining weight but not energy. The heart is a muscle, the one muscle in the body that never rests. Clearly it is particularly important that it has sufficient carnitine to generate the energy needed to maintain adequate blood flow to all the other cells so that they in turn can obtain the energy they need.

When tissues have been starved of oxygen and are then suddenly flooded with it, there is a lot of repair and maintenance to do. The oxidative machinery has, by definition, slowed down and there is now increased activity and therefore increased production of free radicals as this speeds up. For this reason, antioxidant nutrients are important. These include vitamin E, well known for its benefit to the heart, as the Shutes showed decades ago, citing remarkable recoveries from heart attacks of people who were given this vitamin. Other important anti-oxidants are beta-carotene, vitamin A and C and several trace elements such as selenium, zinc, copper and manganese. The herbs ginko biloba and bilbery also have useful antioxidant properties that can help the heart and crataegus (or hawthorn) is a well-recognised cardiac tonic herb.

While vitamin E is extremely valuable to the heart, it

should be taken with caution by people with high blood pressure. It is not that they don't need it; they do, but they also need to give their body time to adjust to its benefits. If you have high blood pressure, you should start with a dose of 50 I.U. or less and build up gradually, monitoring your blood pressure as you do so.

Coenzyme Q 10, commonly known as CoQ 10, is an enzyme involved in the production of energy. It also protects the mitochondria, the energy production sites within the cells, from damage. When muscles are given extra work to do, there can be an initial inflammatory response. The activation of sluggish muscles is obviously a good thing, and this includes the heart muscle if it has been under-functioning, but in the general reactivation process those dangerous free-radicals are generated and the cells, because of their inactivity, have reduced capacity to deal with this. For this reason, the protective activity of coenzyme Q 10 is important for the whole body in general and for the heart muscle in particular.

Note that it is the initial inflammatory damage that coenzyme Q 10 protects against, not the long-term physical damage done to muscles that are over-used and abused, as by heavy physical activity.

There is one problem with this coenzyme. It is very unstable. If you try one brand and don't feel the benefit, look for a better one. You may even want to discuss this with the manufacturers.

While we have focused on a few specific nutrients, the heart is also composed of typical cells and they need all the vitamins, including the B-group vitamins needed for energy production, just as we discussed earlier (Chapter Six). All the tissues of your body need all the nutrients. It is simply that some are required in particularly large amounts in certain situations. So make sure your diet is fully adequate if you wish to protect your heart and have it working for you to the best advantage.

The above suggestions apply to an *underactive* heart that is providing insufficient blood flow fully to nourish the cells and enable them to generate adequate amounts of energy. An *overactive* heart is going to need the same type of treatment to compensate for the excessive stresses on it. So either way, you need to feed your heart with all these nutrients.

Blood Clots

Another factor that can slow down the circulation and thus reduce the flow of oxygenated blood to the cells is the tendency of the blood to form clots. When you have cut yourself and the blood is pouring out, the formation of a clot to stem the flow is desirable. What is not desirable is the formation of clots within the blood vessels in your body, which impede normal circulation. Before actual clots form, a preliminary process occurs in which the platelets start to clump together. Platelets are small entities, much smaller than any of the other blood cells, and their main function is to initiate clotting. A simple test that involves looking at the blood under a good darkfield microscope will show whether or not these platelet aggregations occur too extensively. If they do, something should be done about them.

Prostaglandins are instructional molecules produced within your body. They are somewhat like hormones except they are produced on the spot, act immediately and then break down, whereas hormones are produced by a gland in one part of the body and then travel throughout your system, passing on their message and creating their effect. There are three sub-groups of prostaglandins and the group that is most effective in preventing unwanted blood clots is the Prostaglandin 3 group. These are made from the fatty acids found in fish and so it is important for your heart to include fish in your diet. For the same reason, an EPA supplement is important. EPA, the abbreviation for eicosa-pentaenoic acid, is one of the important fatty acid derivatives necessary for the production of this group of prostaglandins.

It is also important that you cut down on your meat consumption, as meat contains arachidonic acid, the fatty acid that is converted into the Prostaglandin 2 group, and this group encourages the blood to form clots.

Vitamin E is an important antioxidant and works with EPA to help reduce the viscosity of blood and minimise the risk of unwanted blood clots. Magnesium is a helpful mineral and manganese, zinc and vitamin C help catalyse the conversion of the fatty acid into the desirable, anti-clotting, group 3 prostaglandins.

Garlic is also very good at thinning the blood and some trials have shown it to be better than aspirin at this with none of aspirin's side effects, such as damaging the mucosa of the digestive tract and causing ulcers.

Arteriosclerosis

It is not only the heart and the blood viscosity or stickiness that may be involved if you are suffering from cardiovascular problems. There may also be problems relating to the arteries and to their walls. Your arteries carry blood from the heart to the rest of your body. They have muscles along their walls and it is the job of these muscles to relax and contract alternately and thus to send the blood along its way to the capillary beds, from where it later returns to the heart via the veins. These artery walls need to be mobile and flexible for this circulation to occur correctly. However, with age they often become stiff, hardened and less active. This is called arteriosclerosis (or artery walls hardening) and as a result of this process the blood flow is not as good as it should be. This may affect the arteries that supply blood to the heart muscle itself so that it pumps less energetically; it may affect the blood supply to specific organs and tissues, depending on the location of the arteriosclerosis; or it may affect your whole body if the arteriosclerosis is widespread.

Atheromas and Atherosclerosis

Further problems in blood flow occur when the artery walls become thickened as a result of atheromas. These atheromas are formed *within* the artery walls. They are not, as is so often thought, simple deposits of fats and other materials *on* the artery walls. The thickenings can be initiated by a variety of factors including cigarette-smoking and stress. It can be triggered by many other toxins including agricultural insecticides and pesticides, a variety of food additives, and a range of toxic chemicals absorbed into the system, and by free radical damage (hence the need for antioxidants, yet again). We will come back to these shortly.

Ironically, they can also be caused or worsened by the polyunsaturated margarines you are encouraged to eat for your heart's sake. The first step was to encourage you to eat unsaturated rather than saturated fats, reasonably enough. The problem is that the unsaturated fats are generally liquids, like the vegetable oils, and people want a solid spread to replace butter, which is fairly highly saturated. To achieve this, the process of making the oils into a solid was developed. This involves first activating the oils and then hydrogenating them. As a result, they become somewhat more saturated as well as more solid, but still less saturated than butter. However, in the process trans-fatty acids are found and these are the compounds that cause the problem. They reduce the conversion of unwanted cholesterol-rich LDLs to the low-cholesterol and beneficial HDLs. We will consider this in more detail later in this chapter.

People I have spoken to within the margarine industry know about this and have told me they are looking for ways to reduce the amount of trans-fatty acids that are formed during the process. However, they will not put this knowledge into practice until they are forced to, as the trans-fatty acids make the oil more solid and so reduce the amount of hydrogenation required. This enables them to boast of a high polyunsaturate to saturate ratio, a market edge no company is keen to lose.

Atheromas can occur whether or not your blood fat level is high and whether or not you have a high cholesterol level. This is an important fact to remember. If the atheroma then becomes hardened, by the inclusion of calcium, it develops into atherosclerosis. Thus both the arteries (arteriosclerosis) and the atheromas (atherosclerosis) can become calcified and hardened. This is not, however, an instruction to you to eat less calcium. Hardening will occur even if you are on a low calcium diet. Calcium is definitely not the problem, the hardening is a consequence of faults that have already occurred, as we will find out shortly.

Once the atheroma has been triggered by some agent and has started to form, it actually manufactures its own cholesterol on the spot. In addition, it draws in substances from the blood, including fats and cholesterol, even if the level in the blood is relatively low. This is why some of the results and information regarding cholesterol are confusing. A high level of cholesterol does indeed seem to be a risk factor for heart disease (though not for its own sake necessarily, as we shall see). However having normal or low levels is not necessarily a reason for complacency. As you will have realised from the above, the first and most important step is to ensure that you do not initiate atheromas in the first place. The

way to do this is to ensure proper nutrition, a plentiful
supply of antioxidants and the avoidance of the various
damaging factors.

Where cholesterol itself is concerned, it is the way in
which it is transported in the blood that is at least as
important as the total amount present. To understand
this, we need to find out what happens to fat once you
have eaten it, digested it and absorbed it from the intestines into the blood. Normal lipid (fat) metabolism
depends on several factors, including the amount and
type of fat in the diet, the state of your digestive system
and the metabolic capacity of your l. 'er. The main lipids
that you eat are the saturated and unsaturated fatty
acids that make up the triglycerides of food, and cholesterol.

Normal Fat and Cholesterol Metabolism

It is relatively easy for proteins and carbohydrates to be
carried in the aqueous bloodstream and flow throughout
your body. By comparison, it is relatively difficult for
fats to move through this medium. Because of this, and
since you have no nutritional need for fat other than for
a small amount of essential fatty acids, it is a lot healthier
and a lot easier for your body to handle a diet in which
fat makes up no more than ten to twenty per cent of the
calories supplied than when you eat the normal fat-rich
diet of today in which it is common to find that well
over half the calories come from fat.

Almost every time people think about diet and their
heart, they think about cholesterol. There is a lot of
misapprehension about this and, since it relates to your
heart and thus to your energy, a discussion is appropriate. The fear of this substance over the past few decades
seems to have been misplaced. At the same time it is
appropriate to wonder what metabolic errors are occur-

ring if the blood levels of cholesterol do become abnormally high and why this could be a problem. Cholesterol is a large molecule, much larger than glucose, the fatty acids or the amino acids to which the rest of the food molecules are reduced. It has many vital roles to play in the body but when it has finished and needs to be disposed of, there is a potential problem as the cells have no way of breaking it down. It can only be eliminated from your body in the bile, via the liver and gall bladder. The secreted cholesterol then travels down the intestinal tract, some of it (about ten per cent) is eliminated and the rest is reabsorbed. If this route is in some way restricted or blocked, blood levels of cholesterol can rise.

One safe and harmless way to help correct abnormally high blood levels of cholesterol is to improve liver function, (See Chapter Twenty-seven); another is to reduce the amount that is reabsorbed and increase the amount that is eliminated. This can be done by increasing the fibre in your diet. This fibre absorbs some of the cholesterol that enters the digestive tract from the liver and it is lost in the stools.

To get an overall picture of what is happening, we need to consider the way your body handles all the fats that you eat, including triglycerides and cholesterol. Ideally the fat you eat should be unsaturated rather than saturated. In the original caveman diet (Chapter Two) when we ate flesh from animals that had run wild and exercised extensively, we were eating food in which the fat was relatively unsaturated, as it is in ocean fish today, which are also running (or swimming) wild. Now that the meat we eat comes from sedentary animals who have nothing much to do all day but eat and sleep, the flesh we eat is relatively rich in the less healthy saturated fats rather than unsaturated fats. It is worth noting that for the same reason you too will benefit from regular and frequent exercise as opposed to a sedentary lifestyle.

When you eat fat, as we have already seen (Chapters Three and Five), the liver has to produce bile and the gall bladder has first to store and then release it. If your liver and gall bladder are not functioning well, normal fat digestion and absorption will not occur and there will be problems. We have already covered that, but it is worth reiterating. What really concerns us here is the next step. Once the fats have been absorbed into the bloodstream, they go, eventually, to the liver where they are processed, hence the need for a healthy liver.

From here on, the process is somewhat complex. If you are not interested in the details, skip the next few paragraphs and read 'What to do'.

To enable the triglycerides to travel from the digestive system to the liver, they are wrapped up in globules called chylomicrons which contain proteins and cholesterol as well as the triglycerides (fat) you have eaten. To create these chylomicrons, the cells in the walls of the small intestine have to manufacture the cholesterol they need. In other words, *the more fat you eat, the more cholesterol your intestinal wall cells have to make.*

Once these chylomicrons reach the liver, they are rearranged into Very Low Density Lipoproteins or VLDLs, which are made o protein, lecithin, cholesterol and triglycerides. If there is insufficient cholesterol to make these VLDLs, the liver will synthesise more of it. *Again, the more fat you eat the more cholesterol you have to make*, this time in your liver. As they travel throughout your bloodstream, these VLDLs deliver triglycerides to the various cells in your body, either for energy production or, if you have consumed an excess, for storage in your adipose tissues.

Eventually, these depleted VLDLs go back to the liver and are converted into Low Density Lipoproteins or LDLs. They are now relatively less rich in triglycerides and relatively more rich in cholesterol than were the

VLDLs. These LDLs now travel through the bloodstream and deliver this cholesterol to the tissues that need it.

It may surprise you to know that *cholesterol is an extremely important substance and nutrient* (otherwise it is unlikely that it would be provided in the egg for the developing chick, where space is at a premium) and that it is required by a wide variety of organs and cells. It is needed in considerable quantities in the body for the formation of vitamin D, which in turn is required for calcium absorption; it is essential for the production of bile in the liver; for the production of the sex hormones such as testosterone, oestrogen and progesterone; and for the production of the corticosteroids such as cortisone. It is an essential part of the structure of cell membranes, an important component of nerve cells and in high demand within various parts of the brain. It is also essential for the transportation and metabolism of the major group of fats in the diet and the body, the triglycerides, as we have just seen. Cholesterol has many uses and is vital to your health when supplied in the correct form and the correct amount and then, once spent, appropriately excreted from your body.

Back to the LDLs. Once they have delivered their spare cholesterol, these LDLs also return to the liver. By now, the important role the liver plays in fat and cholesterol metabolism should be obvious. When they leave the liver again they are High Density Lipoproteins or HDLs, which still contain some cholesterol, though only a relatively small amount. These HDLs are able to travel through the blood stream more easily than the VLDLs or the LDLs. Their job is to pick up used and unwanted cholesterol from tissues. Remember that, since your cells have no way of breaking down cholesterol, the waste material has to be taken to the liver where it is converted into bile and eliminated from the body via the gall bladder, small intestine and colon. These HDLs are the good guys, picking up and getting rid of unwanted cholesterol and thus helping to avoid a build-up.

The full sequence is:

Chylomicrons → VLDLs (which deliver triglycerides) → LDLs (which deliver cholesterol) → HDLs (which pick up unwanted cholesterol and return to the liver) → bile and disposal.

From this, it is clear that if you have a high cholesterol level and it is in the form of VLDLs or LDLs, you have a problem, since fats and cholesterol are being distributed around your body. On the other hand, if your cholesterol is in the form of HDLs you are far less likely to have a problem as any unwanted or 'spent' cholesterol can easily be picked up and eliminated from your body.

Earlier, you learned that a variety of toxins can cause atheromas to develop. Many of them, including the agricultural chemicals and food additives, are fat-soluble. These are carried in the fat-rich VLDLs and LDLs rather than in the HDLs. So the more VLDLs and LDLs you have, the greater will be the load of toxic, fat-soluble chemicals carried in your bloodstream and capable of initiating atheromas. The longer these VLDLs and LDLs exist before eventually being converted to HLDs, the longer the toxins will circulate throughout your arteries, increasing the risk of atheroma formation.

Clearly, the process of converting LDLs to HDLs in the liver is an important step and one that you want to encourage. Vitamin C is an essential vitamin if this step is to occur smoothly and readily as it acts as a co-enzyme or co-catalyst in the conversion of the cholesterol into bile salt and bile acids.

There is also a somewhat ironic factor that slows this conversion step down, namely the presence of (abnormal) trans-fatty acids in the liver. You will recall that these abnormal fatty acids are made from (normal) cis-fatty acids during the process of converting vegetable oils into margarine. (Do not worry about what cis and trans mean, they are chemical terms and need not concern us.) This means that eating margarine is likely to *block or reduce* the conversion of LDLs to HDLs, the very step you *do* want to occur to reduce your risk of high and unwanted cholesterol. By blocking this step, margarine can actually *cause* your level of cholesterol-rich LDL to build *up*, the thing you are trying to avoid. It is therefore surprising that you have been encouraged to eat margarine at all. Unsaturated fats are fine, and can be obtained from oil-rich seeds and vegetable oils. What you do *not* want is unsaturated fats that have been processed into more saturated fats such as margarine (to make them solid instead of liquid) with the concomitant production of these dangerous trans fatty acids.

What To Do

If you want to avoid atheromas, keep your arteries clear, allow a plentiful supply of blood to course through your body and have plenty of energy, then keep your diet low in fat overall, choose unsaturated fats found in plant foods rather than saturated fats and avoid processed fats such as margarine. By keeping your intake of *fat* low you can reduce the amount of *cholesterol* you make in your body. It is the total amount of fat in your diet about which you should be concerned, much more than the quantity of cholesterol you eat, which, as we have seen, is a nutrient that is vital to the life of all cells in general and many organs or types of cells in particular.

Concerns about cholesterol are gradually being brought into perspective and the fear of it is gradually being replaced by the recognition that many of the ideas were myths. Yet this is not an instruction to go out and eat all the cholesterol-rich foods you want. If you *do* eat a high fat diet and a lot of cholesterol-rich foods and margarine and your diet is low in vitamin C and you consume a lot of the toxins listed above, it is definitely time for change. It is simply that the more important steps are the correction of all the other factors, not simply the reduction of your cholesterol intake. The high blood cholesterol level (as LDL) is a symptom of a problem, not the cause.

Eating cholesterol does not necessarily lead to high levels in the blood. High blood levels are not necessarily dangerous. Forcibly lowering blood cholesterol with drugs has been shown to generate unpleasant and adverse side-effects and to provide no overall benefit to your heart or circulation system. It is perfectly possible to have a heart attack when your blood cholesterol levels are low.

I recall a colleague telling me the following story. A chap went to see his doctor for a check-up, during the course of which he was told his cholesterol level was at the upper edge of normal. He asked what he should do about this and was told to stop eating eggs and come back in three months for a check-up. He did this and found, to his dismay, that his level had risen fifteen per cent. He was then advised to cut out meat, eat margarine instead of butter and reduce the overall amount of fat. At his next check-up his cholesterol level had risen a further twenty per cent. Eventually he was put into hospital for observation and given a virtually fat-free diet. When his blood cholesterol level continued to rise my colleague was called in.

The problem, once recognised, was simple. He had been told what he should not *eat but not what he* should *eat instead. When he had been told to stop eating eggs (rich in cholesterol, it is true, but also rich in a large number of vitamins, minerals and important nutrients such as lecithin), he had replaced these with processed breakfast cereals (refined carbohydrates low in nutrients) to which he had added milk and sugar (an excess of which in the body is converted into fats and then stored). When he had been told to stop eating meat, he had replaced it with pizzas and bread (lots of white flour) and bigger helpings of desserts (sugars). In the hospital, since so much of the standard food was denied him, he had been eating bread and jam whenever he got hungry.*

When this was replaced with a diet consisting of lots of fruits and vegetables, freshly grown sprouts, legumes such as soy, red kidney beans and so forth, plain yoghurt, brown rice, whole grains, fish, a small amount of olive oil and, yes, eggs, his cholesterol level returned swiftly to his starting point and then fell below it, to the lower edge of normal. He was also given vitamin C, to encourage the conversion of VLDLs and LDLs to HDLs, and a full spectrum nutritional supplement.

Keep in mind that because of cholesterol's importance to your body it is fortunate that you are able to make it if there is an inadequate supply. Your liver and the cells of the walls of your small intestine are perfectly designed to make more as it is needed. If the diet contains a lot of cholesterol then less is made; if it contains only a small amount of cholesterol then more is made. The amount made depends on your total fat intake and this is what should be reduced.

What You Can Do

There are a number of nutrients that help to improve your liver's ability to handle fats. These include lecithin, or its precursors choline (found in health food shops as choline bitartrate) and inositol, plus the methyl-donating amino acid methionine, several of the B group vitamins and vitamin C. Several herbs and other plants are helpful, including dandelion, chelidonium, fringe tree bark, beetroot and radish.

Cholesterol reabsorbtion can be reduced by adding to the diet the type of complex carbohydrates that cannot be absorbed – the type commonly, though inaccurately, known as fibre. These include vegetable phytosterols and food sources such as oat bran and rice bran and ground psyllium seeds. Other useful fibre foods include the bran of other grains, soy fibre and the fibre of other vegetables and fruits.

Here are some general guidelines to help you look after your heart. For more information, you should consult some of the books written specifically about nutrition, lifestyle and your heart.

- Eat a low-fat diet, with less than twenty per cent of the calories coming from fat.
- Eat unsaturated vegetable and fish oils rather than saturated animal fats, but avoid margarine.
- Eat lots of vegetables and fruit, making sure you have a high intake of plant fibre.
- Eat whole grains for fibre, nutrients and low-fat proteins as well as their complex carbohydrates.
- For protein, eat fish, eggs and cottage cheese in preference to meats and hard cheeses.
- Avoid salt. There will be plenty in your diet already, if you buy any processed foods at all or if you eat out.
- Avoid tea and coffee.
- Don't smoke. The compounds inhaled can cause atheromas.
- Keep your weight within the normally recommended limits for your height.
- Do aerobic exercise daily for at least twenty minutes at a time. Aerobic exercise means you should be

puffing gently while you are doing it. This shows you that you are needing more energy than usual and so needing more oxygen to burn up the fuel.

- Drink two litres of purified water a day.
- Take the type of general supplement programme of vitamins and minerals that we have already discussed and one that you can feel making a difference to your health, energy and well-being.
- Add lecithin to your diet. It is of great value to your liver which obviously has a major role to play in your ability to handle fats and cholesterol.
- The case for alcohol, and specifically for wine, is dubious. There is some evidence that a glass or two of wine (particularly red wine) each day may be beneficial, but other researchers doubt this. The suggestion is that wine increases your level of the beneficial HDLs, but another indication is that it increases a less common type of HDL and one that is not helpful.

  If you don't drink, then don't. If you do, then you could hedge your bets by sticking to a couple of glasses of good red wine. Good wine should have less sulphur compounds and preservatives than less good wines, so could be less likely to initiate atheromas. Remember however, if you have a *candida* problem, wine is definitely out.

References

[1]Seelig, M., 1989. 'Cardiovascular consequences of magnesium deficiency and loss: Pathogenesis, prevalence and manifestations – magnesium and chloride loss in refractory potassium repletion.' *American Journal of Cardiology*: 63: 4G-21G.

Chapter Twenty

Respiratory Problems

It is exhausting to be unable to breathe properly. We have already seen the importance of the oxygen in the air you breathe. It is the essential ingredient that participates in turning the food you eat into carbon dioxide, water and energy. Only a very tiny and limited amount of energy can be produced if the cells lack oxygen.

For you to produce a plentiful supply of energy easily and on demand, several things must happen. First, you must be able to take in the air smoothly and easily through clear nasal passages. It must then pass along clear and uninfected bronchial tubes, after which it must enter lungs that are able to contract and expand smoothly as you breathe in and out. Then there must be the correct healthy structures within the lungs so that the oxygen in the air can cross over the walls of the lungs and enter the bloodstream on the other side. After that, it is up to the iron and haemoglobin in the bloodstream to deliver it to the cells (see Chapter Nine).

Put another way, there are many things that should *not* happen. Your nasal passages should not be obstructed; there should be no mucus or catarrh blocking the tubes. You should not have hay fever with the accompanying swelling of the tissues which restricts the passageways. Your sinuses should not be infected and generating infected mucus to block the tubes. You should not have bronchitis. You should not have asthma decreasing your ability to relax the lungs and exhale, allowing you no space to breathe in more fresh air. There should be no infections in the lungs and there should be no emphysema. If any of these situations are present, your intake of air and its ever-precious oxygen could be impeded and so your energy production reduced. Not only will these conditions reduce your intake of oxygen, they are also energy-sapping in themselves.

If your nose is so blocked that you have to breathe through your mouth, then even though you may get sufficient oxygen, in total, you will find the effort of talking and mouth-breathing at the same time tiring. Try it for yourself, if you don't already have nasal congestion. Hold your nose and try to have a normal conversation. Imagine what it would be like if you had to breathe like that all the time. In addition, the fine hairs within your nose act as filters.

I have had many children as patients who have been brought in by their parents for a variety of reasons but all suffering the secondary consequences of blocked noses and sinuses. These children are commonly tired or lacking in energy because of the constant physical strain of not being able to breathe through their noses. Sometimes the problem is solved by the elimination of dairy products from their diet. Sometimes full allergy testing is needed with avoidance of the foods indicated.

When you breathe through your mouth, a lot more rubbish enters your lungs than when you breathe through your nose. If the obstruction is physical you may want to consider an operation to restructure your nose and airways. If it is caused by mucus, the solution is less drastic physically, and the results can be surprisingly rewarding.

Mucus and nasal catarrh are tedious. If the sinus cavities become blocked, the problem worsens and if they are inflamed they can be very painful. You may have localised pain over the sinuses themselves and you may develop headaches.

Hay fever can be exhausting. The constant sneezing and runny nose, the congestion and inflammation can leave you feeling that your head is blocked, heavy, trying to break out of itself and refusing to function.

These symptoms not only impede the flow of air and thus reduce your energy. They are also tiring in themselves. When your head is 'blocked' by these conditions, it is difficult to think clearly, to concentrate, to use your initiative, to be motivated or to get things done.

All these symptoms can be avoided. For some people, it is simply a case of avoiding dairy products. Mucus, catarrh, even sinus congestion and inflammation can come about when you drink milk, eat cheese or include other dairy products in your diet. You will recall that milk sugar, lactose, is a disaccharide made up one molecule of glucose and one molecule of galactose (Chapter Five). This galactose is further broken down into mucic acid.

Milk can be a problem for people in at least three different ways.

- Some people, as they grow up, produce less and less lactase. This is the enzyme needed in the intestines to enable you to break down lactose. Without this enzyme, the lactose will lead to diarrhoea and intestinal problems.
- Some people respond to the consumption of milk simply by producing mucus, generally in the respiratory tract.
- Others can have a generalised and systemic allergic reaction to milk. This latter can cause a variety of

symptoms, both physical, such as skin reactions and asthma, and mental/emotional reactions from mild mood changes to full psychiatric disturbances.

It is important to distinguish between the three if you say you are sensitive to milk. They may occur separately. Alternatively, they may occur in combination, for instance you may have a systemic allergic reaction to milk and produce mucus that blocks your nasal passages. Like all allergens, milk can be addictive. I have already said that I have seen grown men cry when told they could no longer drink milk (Chapter Eighteen). Many people, when told this is one of their allergens and that they should avoid it, have tried to argue me out of it, saying they must have it, they need dairy products for the calcium and 'everyone says' milk is good for you. You already know that you can get all the calcium you need from vegetables (just as the herbivorous animals do) and that you get a lot of other minerals as well when you choose this source for your calcium rather than milk. No one, after weaning, has an absolute nutritional need for milk or dairy products. For those who can tolerate them, they can be a pleasant part of the diet; for those that can't, dairy products should be avoided.

If you have congested airways, particularly upper airways, then go without dairy foods of any sort, in anything, for a month and find out what happens. You must avoid not only the obvious sources such as milk, cream, cheese, butter, yoghurt and ice-cream, but also any food containing them, such as margarine (milk solids), cakes and biscuits (butter or margarine), soups and sauces (read the labels, or better still, make your own), many breads and a wide range of other foods, unless you have prepared them yourself and know them to be milk-free. If a simple mucus-generating reaction to the consumption of dairy products is the whole problem, your breathing will improve dramatically. If it does not, there may be other allergies and you should have this possibility checked out.

Dairy products are not necessarily the sole offenders. Harry was forty-seven, a lover of fine foods and good wine. He was also tired. He failed to mention to me the obvious fact that he could not breathe through his nose. He failed to do so because this had been a problem for the past thirty years and he took it for granted. We eventually discovered that he was allergic to moulds (including wines, bread and cheese, all of which he loved) and that when he gave them up not only could breathe through his nose, but his energy increased.

Resolving hay fever may also be a relatively simple matter of having some allergy tests done, avoiding your allergens where possible (environmental and food allergies), and going on an oral desensitising programme. This consists of a desensitising solution, one drop of which is placed under the tongue each morning. This procedure can be done for environmental allergens but not for food allergens: it is too risky and could cause anaphelactic shock, which could be fatal.

Because all of these conditions involve allergies or inflammations it is yet again important to nourish your immune system and provide it with all the antioxidant nutrients.

Asthma is another respiratory problem that can be exhausting. It too can be the result of allergies, both environmental and food allergies. These should be tested for and dealt with (see Chapter Eighteen). Asthma can have other causes too.

In asthma, the problem is not that you cannot breathe in, but that you cannot breathe out. Obviously, if you cannot breathe out and empty the lungs, there is no space available for you to breathe in more air so the problem is still one of oxygen deficiency. However, this recognition of cause leads to a possible solution because it involves the muscles of your respiratory system and the way they function, or fail to function. For you to be able to breathe out, the muscles of your lungs and around your bronchial tubes and the muscles of your chest and chest walls must be able to relax. When they do that, your lung structure contracts and the air is expelled. Another muscular reaction is involved in taking the next breath.

Muscles that cannot relax are often lacking sufficient calcium or magnesium, so if you have asthma, you should consider whether or not you may be deficient in calcium or magnesium. A hair analysis will give you clear indication. Failing this, look at your fingernails. If they have longitudinal ridges, however fine, or if they break easily or tear, you are probably lacking in calcium. Do you get cramps? Do you hiccup? Do your teeth break easily or get cavities? There are many signs that suggest a lack of these two minerals.

Do not take calcium on its own. Take it at least in combination with magnesium and preferably in combination with manganese, zinc, copper and silica as well, so that you feed your total muscular–skeletal system in balance. This suggestion will be somewhat different, of course, if you have had a hair analysis and know just which minerals you need and which you don't.

You will remember that it is relatively difficult for your body to absorb minerals (Chapter Seven), at least by comparison with the absorption of vitamins and the macronutrients. For this reason, you need to do all you can to assist the process. Since vitamin D is necessary for the proper absorption of these minerals, it should be added to your programme, and since absorption of minerals is difficult if there is a lack of adequate stomach acid, this too should be considered, especially by adults.

If you do all these things, if you test to see whether or not you have allergies, if you avoid milk and all dairy products on principal, since they so often cause a variety of problems to the respiratory system, if you supplement your diet with the nutrients suggested above and if you change your diet to include rich sources of these nutrients, you may well be able to throw away your medications and sprays and breathe easily. A word of warning however. Make sure you are healthy and do not need any of the medications *before* you stop using them, or at least before you throw them away.

In addition and if necessary, there are many herbal and homeopathic remedies that can assist in the treatment of asthma. However, we have to stop somewhere and there are many other excellent books on these specific health problems.

Finally, emphysema: what is it, what causes it and what can you do about it? The lungs are not simply hollow balls, like balloons that fill with air and then deflate. If they were, the only oxygen exchange that could happen would be across the walls around the edge of the lungs, and this would be grossly inadequate. Instead, the lungs are filled with aerated tissue, a bit like a sponge or candy-floss. If you imagine the pink of the candy-floss as the cells and structure of your lungs and all the air spaces throughout the candy-floss as the interconnected air-spaces of your lungs, you have a pretty clear idea of the structure. Another way to consider the lung structure is that each bronchial tube, as it enters a lung, divides into two, then into four, then these subdivide into eight, and so on. This subdividing goes on endlessly until the tubes are infinitely fine and surrounded by the thinnest possible cellular structures. All these thousands of cells combine to form a vast surface area, across which you can take oxygen from the air you have inhaled and absorb it into the bloodstream.

What happens in emphysema? Imagine that large fluff of candy-floss. Then pinch a part of it between two fingers. The structure is damaged, the floss sticks together and there is a large air space around it. This is something like the damage that occurs in the lungs when the cellular structure breaks down and with this damage it becomes increasingly difficult to draw in and absorb adequate oxygen for your needs.

Many factors can cause this breakdown. Just as the upper respiratory airways can become irritated by dust, particles, dairy products, allergens and so forth, and secrete mucus in an effort to wash away the offending agent, this may also happen in the lower respiratory tract. Your bronchial tubes are normally kept clear when an irritant comes along, because the mucus-secreting cells secrete mucus to make it sticky and more manageable (just as saliva makes the food in your mouth more manageable and easier to control and swallow) and little hairs or cilia then pass the mucus-plus-irritant back up the bronchial tubes, to be expelled when you cough or 'hawk' and either spit or swallow.

If there is too much irritation and excessive production of mucus, the fine, tiny tubes or bronchioles can become plugged with it. When this happens, the air flow is diminished and the oxygen exchange across the lungs walls is reduced, the lungs lose their elasticity and effective breathing becomes more and more difficult. Many factors can cause this, but air pollution is a possibility and cigarette-smoking is an obvious and self-imposed cause.

The onset of emphysema can be insidious. It may occur gradually. If you do not exercise, you may not notice it happening for a while. If you do exercise, you may gradually find it is more and more difficult to get sufficient breath. This may confuse you if you consider you are fit and should be getting fitter and not more tired.

There are nutrients that are important for the lungs. The mucus membranes need zinc and vitamin A, so add these to your diet and to your supplements. There are indications that the lung tissues of smokers have only twenty-five per cent of the lecithin of the lungs of non-smokers. Whether or not adding lecithin to your diet will change this is unclear, but since lecithin is such a valuable food, and so beneficial for the liver which is sorely tried by all the toxins taken in by lungs breathing polluted air, take it anyway. Add the granules to your muesli, to a salad or to some other food you eat. It has been suggested that you should take at least twenty-five mg of vitamin C for every cigarette you smoke. Some researchers would say seventy-five mg or even more.

Having watched people breathing frantically for air yet failing, because of emphysema, to extract oxygen from it, it seems extraordinary that people are willing to risk the hazards of smoking cigarettes. There is enough pollution in the air of our cities. Sadly, there is not a lot you can do for emphysema once it has occurred.

Take good care of your lungs. If there are problems, treat them, as indicated above. Once you can breathe freely, you will have a lot more energy.

Chapter Twenty-One

Your Weight

Overweight

Being overweight can be exhausting. You only have to see the energy needed and then expended by an overweight person to recognise that. The person who is 20 kg overweight is carrying the equivalent of a large and heavy suitcase around with them at all times, although if their weight has increased gradually they may not recognise this. Not only is there the increased weight to carry, but there is decreased flexibility and ease of movement. This makes bending to pick things up more tiring than it is for a slim person.

If you are overweight, you probably exercise less than you would if you were slim. This is unfortunate, since regular exercise increases rather than diminishes your energy. If you do sufficient exercise to keep fit, you will have more energy, not less, to do other things. If your blood sugar level drops and you feel both tired and hungry, instead of heading for a sugar-rich snack, go for a run. This will increase your blood sugar level, thereby increasing the real energy that is available to you as well as keeping you slim.

Increased weight means increased body fat. We have already seen that fat tissue is the ideal place to store toxins which, when released back into the bloodstream, can cause fatigue. The best way to avoid this is twofold: reduce the amount of toxins you take in and stay slim with limited spare fat stores in which the toxins can be stored.

There are many books on diets. Most of them focus on the physical aspects – what you should eat and when, and what exercise you should do. Some offer very strange ideas and a collection of fads or unhealthy weight-loss programmes; many of them are excellent. Some encourage you to lose weight slowly and others offer crash diets. Above all, you want an eating programme that will allow you to lose weight just as fast, and no faster than, your skin can shrink along with you, so there are no unwanted bags and sags. You also want one that will provide the best of health and that will, on an ongoing basis, enable you to stay slim. I have found in my practice that the best programmes are those in which people stop considering themselves to be on a diet but rather recognise that they have changed their eating pattern for good and that this new way, whatever it is for them, allows them to lose weight steadily and healthily and at the same time is enjoyable and satisfying.

The other aspect of weight loss is mental and emotional and there are books on this too.[1] Many people have unrecognised and unconscious fears and reservations about being slim. Neither they nor the practitioner or person planning the diet for them may recognises them, and yet they can sabotage any weight-loss programme. Since they are operating at the unconscious level, you have to work at the unconscious level to recognise and identify them. This is often a significant personal challenge, yet the rewards for weight, health and energy are often major. Losing weight, if you are overweight, is important and both the physical and the mental/emotional aspects should be considered. If you are tired, then that may be the extra trigger you need to make the changes that will lead to the figure, and the energy, you want.

Lose Weight and Increase Your Energy

When you go on a diet, it is important that you do so in such a way that you are not left feeling even more exhausted. To achieve this, it is essential that you increase your intake of supplements, for many reasons.

- When you lose weight, you are taking in less food and calories than you need and relying on your body fat to supply the shortfall in calories. Your body, particularly the fat you are trying to use up, is a very poor source of nutrients, containing virtually none, so you need to get even more from your diet than before you started, not less.

  For this reason it is essential for maximum health and energy that you take good general vitamin and mineral supplements when you go on a weight-loss programme.
- As you lose weight, you will be breaking down fatty tissues. You will then be releasing at least some stored toxins that were in these fats. You need extra nutrients to enable your body, particularly but not exclusively your liver, to detoxify these toxins in the quickest and safest way possible, so that you have a minimum of adverse symptoms (Chapter Twenty-seven).
- One of the reasons people break their diet is because they get a sudden energy drop as their blood sugar level falls. To make it easier to stay on the diet, it is important to control your blood sugar level and so prevent those energy-sapping, binge-creating drops. In this way you control your appetite and reduce

the incidence of cravings and the sudden desire to eat anything in sight. It is not always willpower you need, often it is improved nutrition. As we have already seen, the B group vitamins, vitamin C, chromium and zinc are important for the proper metabolism and maintenance of your normal blood sugar level.

- If you have food allergies, these should be identified and eliminated from your diet. You now know (Chapter Eighteen) that many people become addicted to their allergens. Thousands of diets have been broken by people who simply cannot resist the craving for endless quantities of one of their allergens once they have eaten even a small amount.
- You want your skin to shrink as you do, not to be left with unsightly wrinkles as the fat inside disappears. A variety of nutrients are important for this, including the fat-soluble vitamins, particularly vitamin E, and the essential fatty acids.

It is worth finding a supplement programme that specifically targets weight loss. If it is successful, it will probably include herbs that help to control your appetite and normalise your blood sugar level and fibre that keeps you feeling full by its sheer bulk when it swells up in your stomach, in addition to all the vitamins, minerals and essential fatty acids.

Your weight-loss programme should include an adequate supply of good quality protein so that you maintain healthy muscles and lose fat, rather than losing healthy protein/muscle tissues and leaving your fat stores in place. Many crash diets and yo-yo dieting patterns ultimately fail because each time you lose weight you are losing muscle protein and each time you gain weight you are gaining more fat. The net result of this is that you are gradually losing your metabolising-calorie-

burning tissue, the muscles, and gaining non-metabolis-
ing-non-calorie-burning tissue, the fat deposits. As a
result, a time comes when you suddenly find yourself
saying 'I used to be able to lose weight easily, when I
set my mind to it, now the weight just won't budge, no
matter how strict a diet I go on'.

There is another reason for including a significant
amount of good-quality protein in your diet. You will
recall that it takes about thirty per cent of the calories
you get from protein foods to metabolise the proteins.
Thus only about two-thirds of the calories supplied by
proteins are actually available for energy or storage,
effectively reducing your calorie intake.

Remember too what we said about carnitine and its
precursors, methionine, lysine and the B group vitamins
in Chapter Five. All these considerations are especially
important when you are losing weight. Lecithin is an
important nutrient at this time as your liver has to
metabolise a lot of extra fat on this programme. For this
reason, your food intake should be particularly low in
fat. Ideally you should aim for foods of which less than
twenty per cent of the calories come from fat.

Not all calories are created equal and it is important
that you eat a lot of fresh fruits and vegetables. Not only
are they rich in nutrients, but they are high in fibre and
in general they break down slowly in the digestive tract
and help you to keep your blood sugar level within the
normal range.

Underweight

There is great emphasis in our society on being slim,
often unnaturally slim. The fashion magazines extol the
virtues of being slim and looking good. The articles on
relationships, keeping yourself attractive and sexy, also
stress the desirability of being slim, for both sexes,

though particularly for women. Many jobs and careers demand a slim figure, from gymnasts to ballet dancers, from athletes to models. Other jobs require that you look good and this is often taken to mean looking slim as well.

The emphasis can be so strong that you follow this edict slavishly. It can encourage you to be unnaturally thin. You need a certain amount of body fat for protection, for warmth and for energy stores. Your sense of self and confidence should not rely on having to have a super-thin figure. If it does, it is your sense of self that needs attention, not your weight. If you are unnaturally thin, it is difficult to have the reserves of energy you need.

Again, there are plenty of books on the subject and this is not the place to take it further. Just make sure that neither an overweight nor an underweight problem is a contributing factor in your fatigue. If you think it is, do something to rectify the situation.

References

[1] Xandria Williams, *Choosing Weight Intentionally*, Simon and Schuster (Australia) 1990, Charles Letts & Co. Ltd (UK).

_____

Chapter Twenty-Two

Other Health Problems Resulting in Fatigue

The health problems discussed so far are some of the main ones that have fatigue as a major or serious symptom. There are many others. There is almost no health problem that does not reduce your energy level.

Infections

Infections, from the common cold to pneumonia, from cystitis to nephritis, and from gastritis to hepatitis, are all exhausting. We have already discussed your immune system and what you can do to support it.

Your Back and Your Bones

A bad back can be exhausting, and often there is little or no need for it. Make sure that your diet provides plenty of calcium *and* of all the other nutrients needed by your connective tissues. We have listed them elsewhere but it is timely to mention them here again.

Certainly calcium is important, since it is the mineral present in the greatest concentration in your bones, but other minerals are needed too, including magnesium. The connective tissues that surround your bones help make up the joint capsule that connects bone to bone, are involved in the connecting of muscles to bones and contribute to the discs that sit between the vertebrae of your back all need other minerals as well as calcium and magnesium, particularly manganese and zinc. Copper, (which you will get from your water supply if the pipes are made of copper) and silica are also important. Vitamin D is important for calcium absorption and vitamin C is essential for all your connective tissues. The gross vitamin C deficiency disease, scurvy, is marked by disintegration of the connective tissues.

Take care of your back while it is strong. Learn to lift things in a way that is both safe and effective. One bad lift too many may leave you unable to lift anything at all. Once you have strained your back, it becomes increasingly vulnerable and the pain of ongoing, chronic back problems is exhausting. I have patients who come into the clinic with their own special cushion as sitting in a normal chair, without the perfect support for their back, has become unbearably painful.

The problem started when we got off all fours and stood upright. The spine is superbly structured for walking on all fours as all our internal organs hang down from it. As soon as we stood upright, things began to shift. With age, this becomes obvious in the pear-shape that develops as the internal organs fall under gravity. You may weigh the same as you did years ago, but your centre of gravity has fallen. We now know that people are taller in the morning, after a night during which their spine was approximately horizontal. By evening, you have shrunk as the gravitational forces have caused your spine to compress on itself. Keep this in mind when you are tempted to make excessive demands on your back.

Any pain is exhausting but a bad back is not only

painful, it also interferes with many of the things you want to do.

Arthritis and Related Diseases

Here you have a combination of inflammation, pain, and reduced mobility. All these can cause fatigue. Arthritis is often caused by, or contributed to by, allergies, so have this possibility investigated. Modern medicine has little to offer arthritics except for anti-inflammatory drugs, painkillers and operations. The natural therapies have a great deal more to offer and should be the first consideration if you feel you are getting or have got arthritis.

I have had countless patients with arthritis who have gone back to playing tennis, or been able to take up gardening again, with all the stooping and bending, who have managed to walk fluidly again instead of shuffling or limping, all because proper care was taken of their condition. So do not give up hope. Find yourself a natural therapist who specialises in this area.

Liver

Your liver has a lot of work to do. It is responsible for hundreds of reactions, all of them vital to your health. It has a lot to do even if you eat a low-fat diet and avoid toxins. It has a great deal more to do if you eat a high fat diet and give it a lot of extra work to do. If you do not take proper care of your liver and at the same time you overwork it, both you and it will be tired. See Chapter Twenty-seven for ways to help your liver.

Kidneys

Kidney problems commonly lead to toxaemia and this can generate fatigue. One way to help maintain healthy kidneys is to drink at least two litres of water, herb teas, fruit juices and other non-diuretic fluids each day. If your kidneys are underfunctioning it is wise to reduce your protein intake to a level just sufficient to replace the muscle protein that breaks down each day. There are many herbal and homeopathic remedies that can help your kidneys.

A herbalist or homeopath will be able to help you determine which is best for you.

Others

Obviously there are other conditions, not considered here, that contribute to energy depletion. Whatever they are in your case, search them out and attend to them.

This section on the various health problems that could contribute to fatigue is not intended to give you a comprehensive view of each problem and a complete guide as to what you can do about it. To do that would make this book too big to handle. This chapter is intended to alert you to the fact that these health problems could be a cause of, or contributing factor to, your fatigue. If they are, then getting the appropriate diagnosis and finding the appropriate therapy to start you on the road to recovery is an essential step in getting your energy back. Do what you can yourself, even if, ultimately, this recovery needs to include consultation with a professional who can advise you on your own specific needs. Correct your health and your energy will almost certainly increase.

PART IV

Burnout, or Chronic Fatigue Syndrome

Chapter Twenty-Three

Burnout

In the first three sections of this book, we have dealt with the type of fatigue and energy-loss that has occurred for decades, even centuries. The type of fatigue that results from poor nutrition, from being generally 'run down', from a variety of health problems and from specific toxins and allergens. This type of fatigue can be remedied by better nutrition, improving your immune system and whatever health area needs attention, and the avoidance of toxins and allergens.

There is another type of fatigue. This has been recognised for many decades but was relatively uncommon until recently. This type of fatigue is severe, so severe that even moving a limb may be difficult. It can be devastating in its severity, is difficult to treat and may have been present for months or even years. It often follows a severe viral infection and is commonly accompanied by severe pains in the muscles and joints. In the 1970s, when I saw the first few cases, the sufferer was often thought to be malingering, no one, neither their friends nor family, nor their doctor or colleagues, being able to believe that exhaustion could be so severe and total.

When these people say they are exhausted, they do not mean that they are tired and need a pick-me-up. Solving the problem is not just a case of telling them to have a good rest, take a holiday, get a few early nights, improve their nutrition and their supplements and everything will be all right. It is a case of total physical and mental exhaustion and it requires extensive and subtle therapy before it can be reversed.

Many names have been given to the condition. Among the first was the 'Royal Free Hospital disease', reported in London in 1955. Since then, names and descriptions have included 'Epidemic neurasthenia', 'Yuppie Flu', 'Total Exhaustion', 'Burnout', 'Post Viral Syndrome', 'Myalgic Encephalitis' (ME), 'Fibromyalgic Syndrome', 'Glandular Fever', 'Chronic Fatigue Syndrome' (CFS), and others. In many ways the saddest and most cruel name applied is 'It's all in your mind' – clearly telling the person suffering the symptoms that they will receive little sympathy or constructive help for their plight. Many cases have no obvious features that put them in any of these categories, yet the person is totally exhausted and *knows* that there is something severely wrong.

Take the case of Matthew. Matthew had been a busy executive in a marketing company. He had always been an energetic person, constantly surprising his friends and his family by the amount of energy he could put into his work and still have plenty left over for his hobbies, socialising and sailing, at weekends. He could

*arrive home at 7.00 pm after a fast day at the office and
be set to go out for dinner with friends and chat till late.*

*Then suddenly his batteries seemed to run down. We
pinpointed the change to the time when his father died;
he described this as one of the largest traumas of his life.
It was as if the steam went out of him. He told me that
he now needed to get to bed by 10.00 pm and that even
so he would wake exhausted. At weekends he would lie
in but seemed to be even more tired when he did eventually get up. He lost interest in his yacht, entertaining
friends exhausted him, his drive and motivation at work
were a thing of the past; it all seemed too difficult,
requiring too much from him. Over the past two years,
he told me, it had become a case of coping, of finding
ways simply to survive the demands made on him, of
doing an adequate job in a career position that no longer
interested him, of earning enough to support his family,
of getting through each day before he could, thankfully,
collapse into bed at night, only to wake tired and dread-
ing the demands of the coming day. He had tried a
holiday and had taken a month off to lie on the beach
but after a day back at work he realised that nothing had
been accomplished. What should he do?*

At the time we called his problem, and that of the growing number of people like him, 'Burnout'. Let's explore
it further. In the concept of Dr Hans Selye (architect, as
we have seen, of the concept of the Stress Syndrome and
author of several books on the subject), Burnout is the
third, and final, stage of stress, the stage of Exhaustion
that follows the Acute stage and the Adaptation stage.
Burnout often starts after a major trauma or shock, a
period of intense hard work with extra demands, or
simply an extended period of living hard and fast or a
severe viral infection. During that phase you thought
you could go on forever. You were in fact living on

capital. Burnout is as inevitable as bankruptcy if this process is continued beyond the danger point.

If you are totally exhausted right now, think back in your own life. Was there a time when things changed? Up until then, life was good, you coped well, you were on top. Then something happened, a major stress or trauma, a serious illness, an exposure to environmental toxins or to medications, or a combination of these. Or perhaps it was more insidious than that, perhaps one morning you woke up and thought 'I don't seem to be coping like I used to, I must be doing too much, maybe it's age catching up with me'. Since then, you may have learned to cope, to struggle on, but you know it hasn't been like the old days. You could be in Burnout. You may need to go back only weeks or months, to pinpoint when it all started, you may need to think back years, you may even have to go back to childhood to find the time when it began. Somewhere there may be a dividing time in your life, a time when things changed and you became a different person. You may feel that you have since recovered, though very often recovery is not complete; rather, you have learnt to cope and to accept the changes.

Burnout can be devastating. It can change lives. It can take a long time to recover and some people never do, simply putting it down to the inevitable effect of age. To deal with it you almost certainly need help.

The Cause

Any kind of stress can cause Burnout. For some people, a single or even a small stress may be all it takes; or one ending of a relationship, one loss of job, one trauma, one disapointment, one argument, may be sufficient, not on its own, but as the final straw to an insidious process that has been happening below your level of conscious awareness. For others, it may take a major stress or trauma, or an accumulation of many stresses piled one on top of the other. It occurs when you have reached your own particular limit.

The trigger for Burnout can be physical. You may have been doing too much. It could be caused by a major change in lifestyle, by a move, by an increased workload or a second job to help pay for the mortgage. Burnout can also be caused by the emotional stresses of someone close to you, or by increased responsibility or demands being made on you. It can result from rejection or a feeling of inadequacy.

Burnout, however, is not caused simply by an overload of stress, either physical or emotional, or a period of suffering from a viral illness. As the story has unfolded over the past twenty years or so, it has become obvious that there are other causes for Burnout or CFS. Many people have related the onset of their fatigue to exposure to toxins; to a time when they took medical drugs, be they antibiotics, the contraceptive pill, steroids or some other type of drug; to a time when they painted their house and continued to live in it and breathe the fumes, or when their home was sprayed against insects; to a time when their office was equipped with air-conditioners and fluorescent lights or when they were subjected to toxins in the factory or on the farm.

It now seems relatively clear that what we are facing in Chronic Fatigue Syndrome is an over-exposure to a variety of toxins, xenobiotic substances, combined with a malnourished and weakened immune system plus an overload of physical and emotional stresses. This combination can be a devastating cocktail.

Inevitably, the medical world has sought a 'bug' that could be blamed for the syndrome, an infectious agent or virus. Many viruses have been implicated, as we saw earlier (Chapter Seventeen), but it seems likely that they

were a consequence rather than an initiating cause of
the problem. They were only able to get a foothold
when the above situations occurred, either singly or,
more probably, in combination, hence the name change
from PVS (Post-Viral Syndrome) to CFS.

The Start

Burnout can start at any age. A baby can be born in a
state of Burnout if the mother was exhausted during
pregnancy; failure to thrive may result. A child can
develop Burnout, and the hyperactive child may well be
in this situation. An adult can develop Burnout at any
time, from twenty years to ninety and beyond. It can
happen to anyone. It can happen to the high achievers,
the on-the-go people who seem to be forever pushing
themselves to the limit. It can also happen to the relaxed
and easygoing. It occurs when you have been pushed
beyond your limits, physically or emotionally whatever
those limits are for you.

It can start suddenly. Some patients come in saying 'I
was fine till three months ago, then I seemed to fall to
pieces'. Or it can start slowly until suddenly you realise
that you are not coping anymore, that everything is
getting on top of you. You may look back and even find
it impossible to pinpoint the start. You may have felt, at
some time, that you were having a bad day, then recognised that several days a week were now bad days,
until finally the bad days became so frequent that you
remarked on the good days when your energy levels
were up a bit.

Physical Symptoms

Burnout is utter and complete exhaustion, not just plain old tiredness. You wake tired, not just once but every day. You may wake with a headache, blocked sinuses, or a stiff and aching body. Getting up in the morning is an effort. Getting dressed, doing the routine chores and coping with the basic essentials of the day is an effort, sometimes impossible. Even putting on your make-up, shaving, finding a clean handkerchief, or getting out of your chair may seem like an overwhelming task, requiring more energy than you have to give. Come the weekend, you decide to lie in and 'recover', only to feel worse when you do get up, and depressed when Sunday evening comes round and you're too tired to go to bed, and flattened by the thought that tomorrow is Monday and you still feel as tired as you did on Friday afternoon.

Although you are exhausted, you may have trouble sleeping. Whereas before you went to sleep easily, slept well and woke relaxed, you may now find that although physically exhausted, your brain is racing and you lie awake for hours, searching for the sleep you know you badly need.

You may have small spurts of energy, start on a task, and half-way through find you can't finish it, you are exhausted again. In Burnout, energy is a short-term commodity and easily lost.

Another symptom develops from the fact that you are not coping the way you used to and do not perform the way you once did. You used to be the busy executive, the family provider or carer; people relied on you. Suddenly everything has changed. You can no longer do this, and you doubt your own abilities. You become afraid of what will happen, overwhelmed by your responsibilities. Your sense of your own competence and ability to cope is challenged. Burnout claims the athlete who rose steadily to a height, peaked, and then some-how just never ran or played as well again; the triathlete who was suddenly too tired to train; the high achiever who left university, worked steadily up the corporate ladder and then suddenly started clock-watching and going home early; the positive leader who suddenly can't make decisions; the promising artist who sud-denly loses creative skill or performing energy; the person you relied on for support and back-up who is no longer there when you need them, but may be needing your help instead.

In Burnout, your weight and your appetite may change erratically. Changes in eating patterns, from per-petual hunger to a lack of interest in food so severe you have to force yourself to eat, can be a sign of Burnout. Sometimes you may feel that if you could only eat enough you would surely find the energy to keep going. At other times, even the thought of planning a meal is exhausting.

Your interest in sex may also go, along with your interest in almost anything, in life itself. Life, in fact, is something to be got through. Ask someone how their day was. If they reply 'It passed', or 'I got through it', that could be Burnout.

Emotional Symptoms

You may feel embarrassed by the situation since it is much easier to have a named disease. You can then say 'Sorry I can't do so-and-so, I have x disease'. Whereas if you say 'I'm tired' or even 'I'm exhausted', others are likely to say 'Join the club' or 'Aren't we all?', not realis-ing that there is a vast difference between Burnout and mere tiredness or exhaustion. Burnout can cause a major loss of self-esteem, more so than any other illness, just because it is so hard to define, recognise and describe.

Since you may have no real idea of what is wrong, you may feel diminished, a lesser person than you used to be. Not able to do or feel as much, having lost much of your interest and drive, you may feel increasingly inadequate. This can be particularly devastating if you are a high achiever who felt secure in the knowledge that you were looked up to for what you had done and what you could do.

The exhaustion of Burnout is such that it leads to major anxiety and distress. There will be frustration and often a sense of guilt, since you feel you *should* be able to cope and to keep going. But your life has been gutted, half the things you used to do are no longer possible. Despair and boredom are the norm; joy, laughter and anticipation have gone. Since the zest and the interest have gone out of life, you may find yourself saying that you need a career change, a new house, a long vacation, a new interest, anything, just to pick yourself up. Yet you can't be bothered; even the thought of organising anything makes you feel tired. It is all too much. Since the present is painful and the thought of the future exhausting, you may find yourself living in the past and concentrating on past glories. Making decisions and commitments becomes difficult. You concentrate more on yourself than on others – you have to, for your survival.

The effect can be devastating on a marriage. If one partner is in Burnout, not interested in sex, too tired to take care of their looks, or to socialise, and instead withdraws into themselves, the effect on the other partner can be imagined. You hear people saying 'My wife/ husband is just not the same person any more, they're not the person I married'. Indeed they're not. However much the person in Burnout loves you, the effort of communicating and demonstrating this is just too great, overwhelmed as they are by their desire to withdraw and to conserve what energy they do have for the absolute essentials.

You may become over-talkative as you try to whip up your energies and stay awake. If you are out to dinner with friends and find yourself dominating the conversation as a means of staying awake, that could be Burnout. Not only children, but adults too can be hyperactive. This type of hyperactivity may be your desperate attempt to keep lashing your body along into activity. Alternatively, you may become very quiet, the effort of marshalling your thoughts and making the effort to talk and become actively involved in the discussion being just too much.

Overall, those suffering from Burnout withdraw into themselves most of the time. For one thing, it is too much effort to be outgoing, there is a lack of spontaneity and enthusiasm; for another, there is the fear of not being able to cope with the demands of others, and the fear that they will find out how inadequate you have become.

Emotional changes include decreased enthusiasm, introversion and increased irritability. If you are around such a person, you may feel they are constantly in a bad mood, or that you must have done something wrong or become an irritation to them. Since there is less communication it is difficult for you to find out what is wrong. It is also often difficult for the person themselves to know what is happening. At work, they may want to withdraw from the team, to work on their own. 'Go away and don't bother me', 'I'll do it myself,' and 'I can manage on my own' are typical phrases.

Because of the occasional and temporary bursts of energy that can occur, these moods may suddenly lighten and you may find yourself talking to the old cheery optimist who has suddenly returned; yet there will be a brittleness, an artificiality to the mood, and soon there will be a relapse as the exhaustion settles in once more.

How People Cope

Admitting to Burnout is embarrassing unless you, and others, fully understand what it is. Since one of the results is fear about coping, you may start putting yourself in less stressful situations. You may change jobs to one that demands less of you. You may turn down assignments that would have once excited you, refuse invitations you would once have enjoyed, find ways of saying no to visitors. Dropping out, choosing the meditative way, retiring early, may all be ways of coping.

> When asked if they are under stress, many patients will answer 'No', feeling that because their life is quiet now, things should be fine. Yet they may still be suffering from the stresses of the past. One patient, Barbara, insisted she should be able to cope, and have more energy now, since things were going well, not like four years ago when she'd gone through a divorce, a career change and financial difficulties. Yet she was still in the aftermath of that stress, still in the Burnout that had resulted from it.

Jennifer told her husband she didn't want to continue entertaining his business friends so much, using the excuse that the home should be a private place. David, a forceful and successful barrister, decided to 'retire early' to write his memoirs. John and Elizabeth did not take their long-promised world tour when John retired; John, in Burnout, decided it was much more sensible to travel in their own country first, yet somehow even that trip was always being postponed. These are all ways of coping with Burnout.

Commonly, there is a ready rationale for the changes you decide to make. You can justify them on the grounds of 'wanting more time for yourself', wanting time to get out of the rat-race, 'to do other things with your life'. Some people say they are moving sideways to give the younger, up-and-coming generation a chance, or letting the children take more responsibility for themselves. Often there are plausible reasons for the changes they are making. But if you really asked the person, you would find that their old zest is gone and they are glad to have a reason to do less.

Food and Diet

It is common to find that people in Burnout eat more. Surely there is a food somewhere that will give them a lift. They may think they 'need' sugar to keep going; they may overeat, gain weight and still feel exhausted. Children in Burnout turn to sweets. The business executive eats bigger and bigger business lunches, increases the alcohol intake, or drinks more and more coffee, looking for a lift. The housewife 'picks' all day long, especially when she's preparing dinner at the end of an exhausting day and looking for the lift that will enable her to cope through the evening.

Digestion is impaired, so it is easier to eat refined foods rather than whole grains and vegetables. There is less stomach acid, so digesting meat and other protein-rich foods becomes difficult. Shopping and cooking require an effort. Thus you turn to junk foods, to easy-to-eat snack foods and quick take-away meals.

Stimulants and Energy

The person in Burnout is constantly looking for ways to find their old energy. Thus it is not surprising that they turn to stimulants. A drink before you leave the office, a couple of stiff whiskys when you get home, increasing your coffee consumption, smoking more – these can all be ways of trying to increase your energy, at least temporarily, in order to cope. These stimulants may well be doing you more harm than good, but at least they are socially acceptable and legal.

The role of chocolate is worth mentioning. People who eat a lot of it often feel that they crave it for the sugar content. In fact, chocolate is rich in phenylalanine, an amino acid that is converted into adrenalin and thyroxin, the hormones, as we have seen, that are produced by your adrenal glands and your thyroid gland respectively (Chapters Ten and Eleven). Thus the first result of eating chocolate is an energy boost from both the hormones and the sugar. However, it also contains copper which will slow down those same glands, so the next step is a drop in blood sugar levels and an energy drop accompanied by a craving for more chocolate to get back to the initial lift. Thus chocolate is bad for people whose copper levels are already high, which is most people, since there is often a ready (and excessive) supply from the water pipes, in drinking-water. There is also, of course, the hypoglycaemic effect that is generated by the sugar intake.

Many people in Burnout turn to harder drugs. If you are caught up in the busy executive lifestyle, if you have to perform because so many people are depending on you, if the stresses and pressures are just too great, you may well turn to drugs to survive. This pattern is common among actors and singers, artists and couturiers, advertising executives and people who have continually to present themselves to a demanding public. Marijuana, heroin, cocaine – these and many other drugs may be used not for themselves, but as a means to enable the person to cope. The uppers are then followed by downers so the person can sleep, and the pattern is established.

Getting the person off the drugs is not the answer, certainly not on its own. If you do persuade them to stop, cold turkey, you may well find the personality changes are startling and that the (seemingly) alive and vital person (maintained that way by the drugs) suddenly shows the real symptoms of Burnout. They needed the drugs to keep going. The answer is to deal with the Burnout so that they no longer need the drugs; then wean them off the drug. People with plenty of energy rarely take drugs, they would be aware of being over-stimulated. If you are tempted to take drugs, you may well be in or heading for Burnout.

There are also the emotional stimulants. You may go from one relationship to another, one project to another, one job to another, you may take up gambling or playing the market, all the time looking for the stimulus, the excitement, the verve, that you hope will give you your old energy back.

Burnout – The Physiology – What's Going On

If you are as tired as this, there must be something going on inside the body that is different from a simple reduction in energy output from the cells. Burnout is not a simple case of the factors we have already considered, of nutritional deficiencies or poor absorption and utilisation of nutrients. It is not a case of some other health problem that can be understood, explained and dealt with as in some of the preceding chapters. There is a distinct difference. It is like bending a piece of flat metal in different directions until suddenly it kinks and a definite bend is formed with structural change. It is now impossible to get it to lie perfectly flat and look smooth. The marks are there, the weakness now exists. It is not just a gradual change but a specific leap. Something has given way and cannot easily be restored. So it is with Burnout.

For us to understand this, it is important to understand the changes the body goes through as it deals with the stresses of everyday life. We have mentioned Selye's work before but it is worth considering it again. You will recall that the body's physiology goes through three stages as it deals with the demands of stress. Firstly there is the Alarm Stage that lasts a short time and enables you to deal with emergencies as the adrenalin is pumped out, the stage where you can perform seemingly miraculous feats such as lifting a car off a road accident victim, hanging on to someone who is falling over a cliff and hauling them to safety. These are all things you could not normally do, but they can be accomplished in the Alarm Stage of the stress sequence. Secondly, there is the Adaptive Stage when other hormones take over and enable you to deal with long-term stress. The thyroid gland is stimulated since, as we have seen, thyroxin controls your metabolic rate and hence the energy your cells can produce. Now that adrenalin has played its role in the Alarm Stage, other adrenal hormones such as cortisone play a role in the Adaptive Stage. Your body learns to adapt to the stress and to cope. This stage can go on for a long time, often for years, possibly for decades. You will recall that I stressed that you *should* be using this time for rest and repair, not assuming you can continue in this way. Eventually, however, the coping mechanism runs out and a new alarm stage is reached; but since you are out of reserves by this time this becomes the stage of Exhaustion or Burnout. The alarm has been triggered but your body has no more reserves on which to draw. This is when you turn to stimulants in a desperate but hopeless attempt to whip up some more adrenalin, generate some energy and keep going. During the Adaptive Stage more and more thyroxin is produced until there are toxic amounts circulating, yet these amounts are still unable to whip the cells into action. As a result, the eyes bulge and the thyroid gland enlarges.

The adrenal gland also enlarges as increasing amounts of its hormones are required. Cholesterol levels are likely to rise; it is produced in increasing amounts because it is the precursor to many of the adrenal hormones (not adrenalin itself, but cortisone, aldosterone and related compounds). If you find your levels have gone up even though you are eating a low-fat diet, do not blame the food you have eaten. Cut down on the stress and your body will produce less cholesterol. Increasing demands are made on the pituitary gland during this stressful time, as it sends out messages to the thyroid and adrenals, endeavouring to whip them to greater and greater action.

With all this activity going on, something has to give, and the ovaries and sex glands get less attention and decrease in function, hence the diminished sex drive. Clearly, this is a sensible way for the body to cope since survival has to come first, ahead of producing more of the species.

The thymus gland, involved in the immune system, is also compromised. Its capacity to function is diminished and you are more likely to come down with infections in stress and Burnout than when you are full of energy. Major illnesses, including cancer and AIDS, are increasingly likely to occur as you become more and more stressed and your immune system is exhausted.

. When the Adaptive Stage has been prolonged to its limit, and the third stage is reached, major changes take place. The adrenals become burnt out and can no longer perform. Greater amounts of stimulants produce smaller results.

In full Burnout, it is common to find that both the

thyroid and the adrenals have shrunk. If even one of these glands does, then mood swings are likely. These can be minor or severe enough to earn the label 'manic-depression'. During periods of adrenal dominance, frenetic energy and extroversion are likely. When the struggling thyroid is dominant, it is less easy to cope; spurts of energy are possible but you are likely to be introverted, depressed and non-aggressive.

The Harmful Effects of Coping with Burnout

You may well feel that this is all very well, that you now recognise there is a reason for the way you are feeling, but that you can't stop, you and your body are just managing to cope, at least at a reduced level, and you will have to continue to cope. Unfortunately, many of the ways the body has of coping with Burnout, while helpful initially, have long-term damaging consequences.

Being able to cope with stresses from the Alarm to the Adaptive phase was helpful for millions of years. During that time, this mechanism enabled us to deal with sudden emergencies, both the daily emergencies of dealing with a wild animal, fighting or fleeing, and the longer-term stresses like a prolonged cold winter. But when the stresses lifted we were, by and large, sensible enough to relax and recover.

The danger these days is that it is all too easy to assume that just because you are coping now you can go on coping, at the same level, indefinitely. You continue to expect the same performance from yourself as you gave in the past. You deny yourself that much-needed holiday. You don't take on extra staff because you would rather save the money and you think you can continue to cope. But the Adaptive Stage is not for squandering; it is there to enable you to cope until you can relax and recover. You should relearn how to do this.

The Twentieth Century

The twentieth century has added new hazards to our lives, in the form of diminished nutrition and increased toxins. You have more to cope with and less resources with which to cope. It is like being caught in a vice. On top of that, there are more and more pressures to perform and you keep going, or else risk being left by the wayside. Few people like to do that, so they struggle on. It's as if every time they get away with extra demands on their body and their mind, they assume they can keep doing it and there will be no price to pay.

Prevention

It is important, if you want to stay well, that you learn to function below the threshold level that could tip you into Burnout. Since it is impossible to know ahead of time exactly what your limit is as an individual, you had better act on early warning signs, no matter how slight. We live in a society that sometimes seems to condemn rest and relaxation, that often suggests you should feel guilty if you sit around doing nothing from time to time, that rewards the person who goes the extra mile, works that bit harder and longer, and makes the extra effort to perform even better. You may want to reconsider your attitude towards this.

Even before you get warning signs, it is wise to consider whether or not your life is balanced, whether or not you have allowed sufficient time for rest and play, for home and family as well as for work and the things you feel you have to do. Are you taking on too much? Are you taking more pride in doing than in being? Have you had a setback and failed to allow yourself time to grieve and recover? Do you pamper the people around you but fail to pamper yourself?

Consider your answer to these questions. Are there some positive changes you could make right now? It is so much easier to prevent the problem of Burnout than to fix it that you should give these ideas serious thought.

Recent Developments

As more and more people began to suffer from Burnout and more study and research was done, certain patterns began to emerged. It was recognised that this type of total exhaustion often occurred after a viral infection and so the name 'Post Viral Syndrome' (PVS) came into use. Then it was recognised that, although common, this is not always the case and so another name was applied – 'Chronic Fatigue Syndrome', or CFS. This acknowledges that however much the other symptoms may vary, the one overriding symptom is fatigue and that it is generally a long-term situation. As this is the name in general usage today, it is the name we shall now use.

References – for more details

Xandria Williams, 'Burnout', *Australian Wellbeing* No.32, 1990 p.69 1989. (Copies available from the author.)

Chapter Twenty-Four

Chronic Fatigue Syndrome – a definition

Let's consider again some of the names that have been given to this condition of total exhaustion. As we have seen, these include 'It's all in your mind', 'Royal Free Hospital disease', 'Epidemic neurasthenia', 'Yuppie Flu', 'Total Exhaustion', 'Burnout', 'Post Viral Syndrome', 'Myalgic Encephalitis' (ME), 'Fibromyalgic Syndrome', 'Glandular Fever', 'Chronic Fatigue Syndrome' (CFS) and others.

'It's all in your mind'

This is a diagnosis commonly made by doctors when they can find no identifiable organism or identifiable pathology such as abnormal blood levels of enzymes, hormones or other substances, and when there is no clear-cut and well-defined group of symptoms. In the case of CFS, as we will soon see, many of the symptoms are vague, though none the less devastating for that, and some of them could be a part of other health problems. Yet it is often found, after testing, that none of these health problems are present in a form that can yet be identified. They are also covert rather than overt, experienced by the sufferer but not necessarily obvious to the observer, and are not easy to 'prove' to the sceptical critic who finds it all too easy to apply the label of 'malingering'.

For instance, your thyroid gland may be underfunctioning but not sufficiently to show up as a clear case of hypothyroidism after the conventional blood tests have been done for the reasons discussed in Chapter Ten. Your iron levels may still be within the normal range, yet you may have a mild case of anaemia; your cholesterol level and heart and liver enzymes may be within the normal range. All this leaves your doctor feeling uneasily that s/he is being taken for a ride. S/he can find nothing that s/he has been trained to recognise as a symptom or clue to a specific named disease or pathology.

This unfortunate set of circumstances has meant that many people over the past decade or so have been told that the problem was 'all in the mind', that they should pull themselves together and get on with things like other people, that they were making a fuss about nothing, trying to get unwarranted time off work or avoid doing things they didn't want to do, that they were hypochondriacs. Many people with the symptoms of undiagnosed CFS were told they were imagining things, were neurotic, that their repeated visits to a variety of different practitioners stemmed from an unconscious need for attention, in the belief that they would only receive attention and care if they were unwell. They may ultimately have been driven to depression and despair and landed up with psychiatrists and on the receiving end of mood-altering medical drugs.

CFS is definitely not 'all in the mind', it is very definitely a very real problem and one that *is* now recognised and *can* be solved.

'Royal Free disease'

This refers to the Royal Free Hospital in London, which was identified many years ago as the common source for a large number of people experiencing the symptoms of Burnout. Many other such sources have since been recognised and even grouped together under the term 'Toxic Office Building Syndrome'. This refers to the fact that many people have developed CFS after working for a period of time in a specific environment, usually an air-conditioned office bathed in fluorescent lights, with chemically-treated carpets and furniture, electromagnetic fields in front of computer screens and a chemical cocktail coming from photocopiers, white board markers and more. If on top of that they suddenly found themselves working long hours, commuting long distances through heavy traffic pollution, eating quick take-away food and relying on coffee, sugar, cigarettes and alcohol for a quick pick-me-up, they may well have developed CFS. The location, the office building, with its grouping of circumstances, may have been the trigger, but the pattern is that of CFS.

'Epidemic neurasthenia', 'Myalgic Encephalitis' (ME), 'Fibromyalgic Syndrome'

These names all apply to the sub-group of symptoms involving muscle pain and fatigue and altered touch sensitivity. However, these names serve no useful purpose and they direct attention towards a subset of symptoms and away from the main problem. 'Encephalitis' is certainly irrelevant as part of the name since inflammation to the brain is not common.

Muscle weakness, often so severe that even holding a book to read is too tiring, and muscle pain are recognised parts of CFS. The pain may only be slight, but even slight pain on a long-term basis, on top of the fatigue, can seem like the last straw. In other cases the muscle pain can be severe. The solution is not to focus on treating this pain, but to focus on and treat the person for the entire syndrome.

'Yuppie Flu'

This refers to the fact that CFS has been common among the new young, career-oriented graduates. They have grown up at a time when their diet and lifestyle have probably been the worst ever in terms of poor nutrition, with a high exposure to toxins and ready drug medication, to say nothing of other social drugs. There is greater competition than ever before for the best jobs and a secure future. At the same time there is great emphasis on achievement and self-fulfilment. All of this puts a large strain on ambitious young adults. Add to all these stresses the frequency of viral infections followed by the antibiotic–*candida* cycle, and it is easy to see how this group of people have tended to develop the problem more than many other groups.

'Total Exhaustion', 'Burnout'

These are at best descriptive terms of the major symptom, total exhaustion. 'Burnout' has helped many people to recognise that they, or a person they know, have a significant problem, that they are not simply 'tired', that they are not alone and are not malingering. Yet it also has a terminal ring to it, seeming to imply that the person has passed their best, that their days of maximum production and contribution are over. This is inappropriate, since the road back to full health may be long and slow, but it is possible. Once you have regained your health, you may rise to greater heights than ever before, with negligible risk of relapse provided that the causes have been identified and eliminated and that you take

much better care of your health than you have done in
the past.

'Glandular Fever', 'Post Viral Syndrome'

CFS often, but not always, follows on from a period of
viral infection, often EBV or CMV, as we have seen. Yet
the virus is not the original cause of the problem. It is
not the prime, triggering factor, though it may indeed
be the final trigger that tips you over into full CFS. It
may also be one of the first easily-identified and labelled
signs. As we have already seen, you do not succumb to
a viral infection if your immune system is operating at
full capacity (and provided there is no genetic problem
that weakens this). How else do you explain the fact that
some people get colds in the office when others don't,
that some children avoided chicken pox (in the prevacci-
nation days) even when the rest of the school was
coming down with it, and that many sexually-active
partners of people with AIDS are not themselves HIV-
positive? You do succumb to viral infections if your
immune system is compromised, if your total nutrition
has been inadequate or if you have been overexposed to
toxins.

The virus is a common, though not essential, part of
the syndrome. You may have had Glandular Fever, and
may still show signs of this when blood tests are done.
Yet CFS goes beyond this. You may have had some other
viral infection, but the treatment involves more than
dealing simply with a virus.

'Chronic Fatigue Syndrome (CFS)'

This has come to be the most commonly used term for
the condition. Like 'Total Exhaustion' and 'Burnout', it
focuses on the exhaustion aspect of the problem. By
adding the word 'Syndrome', it implies that there are

a group of symptoms and that the problem is a real, identifiable entity. It takes it away from the realm of an amorphous group of symptoms, varying from individual to individual and easily passed off. It is a case of 'unite and rule' rather than 'divide and conquer'. By uniting all the symptoms together in a Syndrome and calling it CFS, many sufferers have found some firm ground in a shifting mass of generalised health problems. The term has also made it easier for practitioners to focus on it as a total entity and look for the possible causes, mechanisms and treatments. Yet the name is sufficiently loose that we can continue to be open-minded and not claim that the symptom picture is carved in stone and you either have it or you don't.

Even though it is likely that the problem has been around for over a hundred years, possibly first labelled 'hysteria', there is a lot we still have to learn about it. It is probably even true to say that the syndrome is still developing as we further manipulate our food supply, add more and more xenobiotic chemicals (toxins) to our environment and override more and more frequently the capacity of our delicate biological systems to withstand the changes brought about by high technology.

New Names

If a new name is to be coined for this condition, it should, in my view, convey the real sequence of events that we now believe is occurring. This is (a) over-exposure to toxins; (b) under exposure to good nutrition; and (c) a failing immune system; all leading to (d) increased susceptibility to viruses, candidiasis, allergies and total exhaustion; (e) reduced ability to handle the stress people are experiencing; and (f) a host of symptoms consequent on this, including but not limited to painful joints and muscles. In many ways, CFS is the result of our body's inability to keep up with the environmental changes we are imposing upon it. Until a name is developed taking this into account we will stick to 'CFS'.

Definition of CFS

CFS, caused as it is by a variety of factors – physical and emotional stress, a weakened immune system, inadequate nutrition and an overload of toxins – is difficult to define. There is no single organism that causes it that might have enabled modern medicine to give the condition a name and prescribe a drug or group of drugs for its treatment. There is no specific group of symptoms such that, if they could be checked off and sufficient of them found to be present, the diagnosis could be made and if absent the diagnosis could be ruled out. CFS is a much more complex situation than that and the diagnosis is usually made on the total history of symptoms, environment and related factors. We need some sort of working definition, but it is important to observe what is developing and pay attention to it, rather than to ossify the syndrome in a definition based on the existing set of symptoms, since it is highly likely that symptoms will continue to change and develop as our environment continues to change and overwhelm people's bodies and their relatively fragile biology. At the same time it is important to distinguish between serious fatigue and tiredness on the one hand and full CFS on the other, as we shall see as we explore what has to be done to correct the situation. By keeping the definition open, we allow for the possibility of recognising development of the syndrome. With the definition below, we also have the opportunity to recognise the early warning signs and start treatment before it develops fully.

Currently, the following criteria are used to identify people with CFS:

- Long-term chronic fatigue of at least six months' duration and following even minor exertion.
- Fatigue that is not improved after rest.
- Confusion, poor concentration, inability to think clearly.
- Poor memory, especially short-term memory.
- Mood changes, elation and depression, irritability and frustration.
- Headaches.
- Difficulty with normal sleep patterns – insomnia and falling asleep during the day.
- Muscle and joint pains.
- Increased incidence and severity of allergies and increased incidence of infections.

All these symptoms may not occur at once; you may skip some of them altogether, though that is not likely. Their severity will not remain constant. You will have good days and bad days, good weeks and bad weeks, even good months and bad months, and, if nothing is done to resolve the problem, good years and bad years. In fact, some of the good times may last so long, you may not relate the next bad phase to the previous problem. You may have assumed you had got over one bout and now a new one has started.

A likely scenario is as follows:
You probably ate badly. Even though you may have thought at the time that you were eating a well-balanced diet, that you were eating plenty of fruits and vegetables and only sinning on junk food occasionally, in the light of the preceding chapters you may recognise that you were not eating well.

You may have been exposed to a variety of toxins or xenobiotic chemicals. This too is hardly your fault. Unless you study the subject deeply, it is all too easy to fail to recognise both the existence of xenobiotics and the quantity you are absorbing. After all, you were only doing what everyone else did, what television and advertising exhorted you to do. You used the sprays, installed the air-conditioning and central heating, and so forth. You were also exposed to a variety of biologically-challenging physical factors: watching television, using the computer, flying in aeroplanes, commuting in traffic or on polluted public transport.

You gradually became run down, but you coped. There were a variety of stresses, but you overcame them or dealt with them as you were expected to do both by those around you and by yourself. You got on with what you had to do.

You had the various vaccinations, starting with those your parents foisted on you as a baby and over which you had no control and finally having a regular flu 'shot'. There is evidence that all of these interfere with the normal functioning of your immune system. You may have had the occasional infection. One or two colds or bouts of the flu in a winter is generally considered to be fairly normal, yet they may have been signs of a weakening immune system. You took antibiotics from time to time as they were deemed to be necessary.

Somewhere along the line you reached breaking-point. Your body could no longer cope with the stresses imposed. The final straw might have been a major emotional stress, or even a relatively minor one. It could be an illness picked up on an overseas holiday or a bout of food poisoning. It could be just one more course of antibiotics, starting on the contraceptive pill or experimenting with a social drug. It could be a wild night out and an overindulgence of alcohol (yeast-rich beer or wine), or a bout of thrush.

The final factor or causative agent is not the major culprit. You finally succumb not to any one challenge but to the combination of all that has gone before. You may be able to eat bread and cheese and drink beer to your heart's content on holiday, but be acutely sensitive to yeast when its effect is combined with the pollution of the city. You may have food allergies and have to avoid them strictly but be able to get away with eating them if you are relaxed and don't watch television. You may fall asleep each evening if you do watch television but be alert and full of energy if you do something else. Don't be too quick to put this down to the nature of your activity, it may be the effect of the television. It is often the combined effect of the different challenges and the different levels of your nourishment and resistance combined that counts. If the odds stack up in your favour, you feel OK. If they don't, you succumb.

What do you succumb to? It may indeed be a virus. You may get a severe bout of flu from which you find it surprisingly difficult to recover. You may get glandular fever. You may become exhausted, feel wiped out and wonder what has hit you. Be that as it may, when you finally develop CFS you will know all about it.

It can happen to anyone. It can happen at any age, even to children. The additional perceived stresses of teenage years, exams and career challenges, can trigger it. It can happen in early adulthood. It can happen at the height of your happiness, after you have married, been on your honeymoon (flying, foreign foods, different drinking water), moved into your new home (lots of new man-made fibres, plastics, polishes and varnishes degassing), and settled into a different routine (stress). It can happen when things go wrong, when the unexpected baby arrives, when you have to give up your old life and stay at home, when there are money worries, or you divorce. It can happen when the children leave home and suddenly there seems to be nothing to do. It can happen at any time, in any place, at any age and under any conceivable circumstances.

Prevention is very much easier than cure. This is always true, and particularly true with CFS. So do all you can to avoid it. Reread this book to this point, heed all the warnings, do whatever you can to minimise the risks.

If it has already happened, do not despair. There is a lot you can do to correct the situation. It may not be as simple as correcting plain old fatigue, even long-term common fatigue. It will involve a lot more than making a few small improvements to your diet and lifestyle, taking a few supplements, avoiding your allergens and reducing the stress in your life. However there is a lot you can do and it is certainly possible to recover your health, energy and well-being. In the following chapters you will find out how.

Self-check Questionnaire

As you now know, there is no simple definition of CFS. If you are wondering whether you are simply tired or are in fact suffering from CFS, check out the list of symptoms below. In general, the more symptoms you have from this list, the more likely it is that you have CFS. If you are in doubt, talk with a professional who understands the syndrome. If you cannot findone, you may simply choose to follow the treatment pro gramme anyway, since it does lead to improved energy and health, even if simple tiredness is your problem.

Tired

You feel bone-weary or exhausted much of the time.

You feel that, slowly or suddenly, you have had to slow down.

You can no longer cope with your old lifestyle and speed.

Small things you used to do casually and easily now seem to be an effort.

You start projects and then feel too tired or lacking in motivation to finish them.

It takes you all your time to cope with the bare essentials.

You can pinpoint the change to a particular stress.

You have had a period of major stress(es) in the past and relatively close to when all this began.

You say of the day 'I coped', 'I got by', 'I managed'.

You find yourself saying 'I can't cope', 'It's all too much'.

Sleep/rest

You experience insomnia although you feel tired.

You wake up tired.

You often wake up with a headache.

You wake with respiratory problems, sneezing, sinus congestion.

You wake with muscle and joint aches and pains.

You have to drag yourself out of bed in the morning.

You have trouble getting going in the morning.

You find that rest or a nap does not help.

You take a holiday and find you feel no better a week later.

Mentally

You have become confused or vague.

You have difficulty concentrating.

You have trouble finding the words you want.

Your memory is poor, especially your short-term memory.

You have difficulty concentrating.

You feel 'woozy' or as if you are suffering from a hangover.

Emotions

You are less optimistic and positive than you used to be.

You are generally pessimistic and depressed.

You get more irritable than you used to.

You are anxious and worry over small things that used not to bother you.

You are more withdrawn than you used to be.

You find you are tending to live in the past.

You feel frustrated.

You have lost your self-esteem and self-confidence.

You now feel guilty that you are not the person you once were, that you are letting yourself down.

You know you are not well but can find nothing specific that is wrong with you.

You feel embarrassed by this and wonder if you are becoming a hypochondriac.

You wish you had something wrong that could be named and dealt with.

Lifestyle

You have recently swapped career path or plans to something less strenuous or demanding (even if for a very good reason!).

You now avoid situations you once used to enjoy.

You avoid social gatherings and dealing with people.

Recently you have either lost or gained weight.

Your appetite has changed recently.

You find you are craving for certain foods, hoping they will give you energy.

You get indigestion and heartburn.

You now find meat hard to digest.

Interest
You are less interested in sex than you used to be.
Yet you possibly search for more relationships, looking for stimulation.
You have lost interest in your looks, your home, office, car, etc.
You are less interested in almost everything.
Sometimes you find yourself talking excessively to hide your exhaustion.
You make occasional frenetic efforts to compensate.

Stimulants
You drink more alcohol that you used to.
You smoke more, or have recently taken up smoking.
You drink more tea and coffee than in the past, hoping for the energy lift they used to bring.
You crave chocolates.
You are considering or have used other drugs.
You have tried vitamins and found they worked but only for a while.

Others
You experience severe and chronic pain in your muscles and joints.

Chapter Twenty-Five

Chronic Fatigue – Treatment Rationale

The treatment for CFS has to be based on the under-standing we have already developed as to how the prob-lem has come about. In some ways it may seem similar to the treatment of fatigue given in earlier sections. It must include those treatments wherever they are appro-priate, but it also has to go beyond them. On their own, and applied one or two at a time, those treatments will not work if you have passed over the boundary from fatigue, low energy and general tiredness, even exhaus-tion, into Chronic Fatigue Syndrome.

In this chapter, we will be looking at the background and rationale for the treatments. Detailed treatment will be described in the following chapters. However, you will find that you are often referred back to the chapters we have covered as they become the next step in treat-ment of your CFS.

Recall the way CFS is thought to have come about. Essentially, it is caused by poor diet leading to a variety of health problems that eventually overwhelm your body in general and your immune system in particular, and on the other hand it is caused by an overload of toxins, pollutants, allergies and medical drugs such as antibiotics and hormones leading, often via candidiasis,

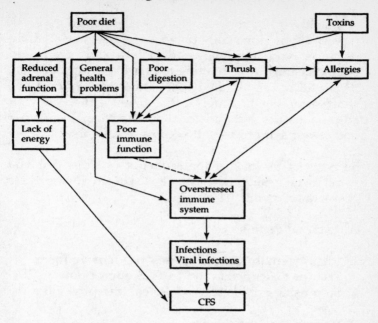

to further and excessive stress on this depleted immune system. As a result of all these steps, you are easy prey for bacterial and viral infections and, since you have few resources left, the situation becomes chronic and exhausting (CFS). It is critically important, as you go through the treatment, that you keep this scenario and concept in mind.

To reverse this process, you have to go back to the start, correct the first steps and work with your body and your environment as it progresses along the flow chart. If you try to work randomly with some of the intermediate steps without resolving the basics, the treatment will not be satisfactory. If you work on the diet and the 'Internal Health Factors' but do nothing about the 'External Factors', or if you change the 'External Factors' but do nothing about your 'Internal Health', it will be like trying to walk with one leg hobbled. Nor will it work if you don't fully unblock the flow lines – if, for instance, you improve your diet (and even add supplements) but do nothing to improve your digestion, there will be only limited benefit and even that may be short-term. If you mobilise the toxins stored in your adipose tissues but fail to eliminate them from your body, your symptoms will become even worse.

So now let us look at the sequence of steps that you need to take and that will be discussed in the three chapters following.

A. External factors

1. Identify environmental causes and remove them.
2. Test for toxic metals and treat as appropriate.
3. Stop using antibiotics and the contraceptive pill.

B. Internal health – basics

1. Treatment of the digestive system and repair of the intestinal mucosa.
2. Detoxification of your system and liver support.
3. Diet and nutritional support – vitamins, minerals, essential fatty acids, amino acids, other nutritive factors – with special emphasis on an antioxidant programme as prevention against both the toxins themselves and your increased metabolic activity as you reactivate relatively dormant systems.

C. Possible associated health problems

1. Treatment for candidiasis and elimination of other unwanted organisms.
2. Testing for, avoidance of, and treatment for allergies.

3. Checking for and treatment of any other existing health problems (Part III).
4. Immune therapy.
5. Endocrine therapy.
6. Improve blood circulation and lymphatic drainage.
7. Sleep therapy.
8. Mild exercise.

C. Mental changes

1. Possible psychological treatment.
2. Cognitive therapy.
3. Stress management.

General

As in all health situations, it is important to make a correct diagnosis. However it is not always easy to diagnose CFS and to differentiate it from general fatigue. This would leave us in a quandary as to treatment were it not for the fact that many aspects of the treatment for CFS are also appropriate as prophylactic measures and all of them are conducive to overall good health and improved energy. If you are simply tired, rather than suffering from full CFS, then the treatment may be more rigorous than is essential for you; however, it will do absolutely no harm – it will improve your health and future make CFS almost impossible, as long as you maintain some of the general changes you have made.

For this reason, if you suspect you are suffering from CFS, if you have been tired for a while and nothing seems to help, your health and your energy will almost certainly improve if you follow the above steps.

Inevitably, the treatment programme for CFS prescribed by a practitioner will be more individual than the one described here. There may be aspects of an individual person's health when they have CFS that makes some of the above steps more important and appropriate than others. However, the general guideline above and the procedures described in the following chapters will make a positive difference to your health if followed thoroughly.

Time

It is important that you understand the severity of CFS as opposed to general fatigue. It has not occurred suddenly. It may seem that way to you; you may feel you were all right until last week, last month or last year and then suddenly you collapsed, your body gave out, and you had what has since been diagnosed as CFS. The last precipitating event may have been a virus, a vaccination, an overload of stresses in your life, but remember, this is just the last precipitating event. If you had been fully and totally healthy, these factors would either not have happened or would not have precipitated you into CFS.

Your current state of health is a consequence of *all* the things you have done in the past. The recent past is particularly important but the distant past can have an effect. I have worked with people with CFS who had multiple courses of antibiotics as children or teenagers and whose health has slowly, almost imperceptibly, deteriorated since then, until 'suddenly' they become aware of problems.

For all these reasons, it will take time to fix the problem. If you are one of the lucky ones – if your CFS is mild and you have only been suffering with it for a short while – the treatment may be rapid and the response good. However, if CFS has been a problem for you for many months or even years, the recovery process may also take months – not as many months as you have had the problem, but still several months. But do it, it will work, and in a few months or a year's time you can be a fully functioning person again.

A Final Word of Warning

When you have been through CFS once you should be careful not to push yourself that hard ever again, otherwise it could recur and be even more difficult to treat the second time around. This does not mean that you should continue to treat yourself like an invalid. It does mean that you should continue to avoid the toxins, look after your digestive system and take the appropriate supplements.

Chapter Twenty-Six

Treatment A – External Factors

Eliminating Toxins – Environmental Steps in the Treatment of CFS

Even if you are currently healthy, it is prudent to remove from your environment as many chemical and physical hazards as you can. Only you can decide whether it is worth the trouble of giving up oven and other kitchen sprays and using less volatile cleaning agents in order to reduce your risk of future poor health and CFS. Only you know whether you are prepared to reduce the toxins in your diet or risk the health consequences that could result. Only you can decide to give up smoking, drinking coffee and consuming excessive quantities of alcohol. It is up to you whether you use a water purifier or are willing to accept the consequences of being subjected to the toxins in your tap water; or whether you are willing to change your saucepans from aluminium to stainless steel or risk the possibility of senility.

What is important is that you take some responsibility in this process and ensure that if and when you get sick in the future, you will deem it an acceptable consequence of the changes you chose not to make in your lifestyle in the past. It is your responsibility to educate yourself, not the responsibility of others. Patients often say to me 'If this food additive is bad for you, why do the manufacturers use it?' It is not the manufacturer's job to provide you with good nutrition; it's your job to see that you are well-nourished. The manufacturer's brief is to run a successful food-manufacturing business and make a profit for the owners or shareholders. They will put in the marketplace whatever they are allowed to and whatever will make the most profit. If people choose to buy quick and easy processed and packaged foods instead of the less processed basics, then the manufacturers will produce them. If people choose to buy white bread, or 'brown bread' made to seem like real wholemeal, then that is what the bakers will bake. If people choose to eat high-sugar lollies and eat strong-tasting and brightly-coloured ice-cream with dozens of additives, rather than the natural variety, then that is what the makers will make. Food processing is done under the guidance of food technologists, who generally do not study nutrition.

Governments are not perfect either. You know that they are made up of fallible people. You also know that they are elected for short terms and often given portfolios on subjects about which they know relatively little. The Health Secretary almost certainly knows nothing about the biochemical and nutritional characteristics of food chemicals, yet s/he may ultimately be responsible for decisions as to whether or not certain additives, pesticides or processes are permitted, and may be susceptible to the influence of multinational companies.

What is certain is that it is *you* who will suffer if you allow yourself to be exposed to and to consume the toxins, not the authorities. You should therefore do all you can to be as informed as you can be about what you put onto and into your body and about the environment to which you are willing to expose yourself.

If you are suffering from full CFS, this avoidance of

toxins is particularly important and it may be essential for you to remove all of them even if this does cause some major changes and difficulties in your lifestyle. You may have to do this at least for a few months, possibly for a year or two.

The home is usually the place with the greatest number of toxins. Refresh your memory of these by rereading Chapter Eight. Start with your bedroom and bathroom. Do you really need all that make-up or all those after-shave lotions? You may find you can change from either high-priced fashion-label cosmetics, or low-priced cheap ones laden with cheap chemicals, to ones made from plant oils and other less harmful ingredients. You may find you have to exchange the perfumes you have been using for essential oils. Essential oils smell nice and have the added benefit of healing. If you must use hair spray, use one with a pump action rather than a chemical propellant and don't breathe in the fumes. You may find you have to give it up all together.

Check your bedding. If you have allergies to dust mites and house dust, you may benefit from special sheeting and pillow covers that reduce your exposure. Eliminate fluffy toys and fluffy covers. It may even be necessary to remove carpets and have naturally-polished bare boards. Rather than open display shelves that can gather dust, have glass enclosed shelves.

The kitchen is often a lethal cocktail of chemicals. Throw them all out. You can get simple soaps or organic cleansers to wash the dishes with. Buy organic fruit and vegetables. If you can't, wash them in a dilute solution of hydrochloric acid and rinse it off thoroughly. Any trace residue of the acid will do no harm as that is the acid you have in your stomach anyway. Check all your foods, read the labels. You may be in for some surprises but the changes you make will pay dividends.

Most patients tell me they can't make all these changes

at once. If you have CFS and want to get over it badly enough, you will make them. Otherwise, it's a bit like knowing what will make you feel better but deciding you only want to get better slowly. Who would make that decision? The only reason there can be for not making the changes rapidly and thoroughly is that you don't believe the information. That is why I have gone to such pains in this book to give you as much detail as possible. Gather more information, talk to people who have recovered. Read more books, consult more people specialised in the treatment of CFS. If you are still not convinced, make small changes and hope for the best, though even this has its drawbacks. Small changes may not be enough to make a significant difference and as a result you may give up, disheartened.

If you protest that you have your family to think about and you cannot put them through the same treatment, stop and think. It is your environment and diet that has had a major input to your health. Even if the other members of your family are still healthy, or relatively so, they may be heading in same the direction as you are. What is good for you as the treatment for your CFS is also good for them for the prevention of CFS and other health problems.

I recall a family where all the members were tired, though none of them thought it worth making a fuss about. The mother had CFS. They decided to do the job thoroughly together, both to help her and as a preventive programme for the rest of them. They threw everything out that wasn't 'natural' – this is a somewhat loaded term and often hard to define, since many toxins are 'natural', but they knew what they meant. They got rid of the alcohol, the tea, coffee and soft drinks. The husband threw out his cigarettes. All the junk food went – mostly to their neighbours. Then they went to the organic food markets and the health food shop and stocked up. Some of the meals they tried to concoct with these new ingredients were a bit unusual, as they put it, but they soon learned new recipes. They emptied the kitchen cupboards of all the cleaning materials and sprays and bought an organic cleanser but, as they said, now they were eating less fatty foods, the oven and plates were a lot easier to clean anyway. In the end, they also pulled up the carpets and reverted to polished floors and Persian rugs which they could beat outside each day. The result, they said, was incredible. None of them had felt so healthy and energetic for a long time and the mother rapidly got over her CFS.

Get yourself a water purifier, one with a reverse osmosis membrane and a pre- and post-filter. You do not need to invest a lot, nor have an expensive one built into your plumbing system. You can get neat and simple ones for around four hundred dollars or two hundred pounds. The saving, compared to buying bottled water, will pay dividends, and because, once you have bought the purifier, the pure water is free, you will use it for everything from boiling rice to cooking vegetables, from making soups to hot drinks, as well as simply for drinking cold. Not only will this reduce your toxin load but it tastes so good, compared to tap water, that you will drink a lot more, to the benefit of your kidneys.

Decide if you really need to watch so much television. If you do, then at least sit a lot further away from it than before and turn it at an angle so you are watching it from the side instead of straight ahead.

Park your car in such a way that the exhaust is directed out at the street and not into the house. Mow the lawn, if you can, with a push–pull lawn mower rather than one that adds more fumes to your environment. It may take longer but is good exercise.

Check your laundry, the soaps, bleaches and fabric

softeners you use. Check your clothes too; you may find that you react to some fabrics.

As you go round your house, you will find other alterations you need to make. Make them, in the interest of your health and energy. Then do the same at work, as far as possible. I had one patient whose desk was in front of the air-conditioning unit and under a strip of fluorescent light. By rearranging her allotted work space and moving her desk, she was able to start her recovery. Get out at lunch-time; the fresh air may not be all that fresh, but it is better than the environment in many offices. If you work in a situation where there are industrial chemicals, find ways to minimise the amount you inhale or that gets on your skin. Wear a mask. This may be a nuisance, but lung disease and CFS are much more than a nuisance. Keep the windows open and the space well-ventilated.

Check the rest of your environment. It is impossible in a book like this to describe everything you may have to do. Some of these suggestions may seem a bit extreme. Having CFS is also extreme and will continue to be so if you do nothing. But as one patient put it, 'It makes you realise just how many chemical and possibly harmful substances we are exposed to'.

Allergies

Allergy testing is essential if you have CFS. If you are simply tired but do not have CFS, you may want to consider whether or not you have sufficient symptoms to make allergy testing essential. But as we have already seen, it is a lot easier to treat tiredness and other isolated symptoms than full CFS. So many people do have allergies yet don't have obvious symptoms that if you have CFS you cannot afford to leave any stone unturned and allergy testing is a very important stone.

It is important that you test for allergies at the beginning of the treatment, before you start on the programme that follows. If you do the tests now, while all the foods you commonly eat are still a part of your daily fare, the tests are more likely to be accurate and to detect your allergens. If you do allergy testing after you have been fasting, or avoiding foods to which you think you react, the tests are less likely to be accurate and you may show up as negative to these foods even though you are actually allergic to them. If you have already been avoiding certain foods, eat them a few times now, at the very start of the programme and before you have the tests done. Don't use this as an excuse to delay starting the programme; one meal of the common toxins is enough. A pizza is a good challenge to include as it contains so many of the common allergens: yeast, tomato paste, anchovies, mushrooms, salami (moulds and yeast), flour (wheat), cheese (dairy products) and tomatoes.

Another reason it is wise to do allergy testing at this time is that once the programme starts you should be taking vitamin C but you should avoid taking high doses of vitamin C supplements for a few days before doing allergy testing. The reason for this avoidance is that vitamin C helps your body to cope with allergens and reduces the reaction. This is obviously valuable if you are trying to minimise the symptoms but unhelpful when you are trying to identify everything to which you react. Later, once the programme has started, you do want to be taking vitamin C and without interruption.

Toxic Metals

Have a hair sample taken and send this off to a laboratory that specialise in Hair Mineral Analysis. Many metals are toxic. Earlier (Chapter Eight), we spoke of analysing a hair sample to evaluate mineral levels and that this test can be used to determine both the level of essential minerals and the level of toxic minerals. There we also covered toxicities, their sources, and the symptoms they can cause. If you are suffering from CFS, it is essential that you rule out the possible adverse effects of any of the toxic minerals commonly encountered. Having a hair sample analysed will not only give you information about toxicities but also useful nutritional information, useful ratios and information about some of your glandular systems (Chapter Seven).

Once you have determined that you have high levels of any of the toxins, find the source. This may be obvious, such as lead from traffic fumes, aluminium from antacids or saucepans, etc, or it may be less clear. Either way, it is important that you do all you can to recognise the source and then eliminate that source from your life. The next step is to take whatever nutritional steps are required to minimise the damage the toxic metals can do and eliminate the existing toxins from your body. Detailed information on this will be given either with the report or by the health care practitioner, naturopath, doctor or chiropractor who has organised the testing for you.

Rest assured that there is a great deal that can be done. A variety of nutritional minerals, can protect you from some of the toxins. We have already mentioned the benefit of calcium and zinc in relation to lead toxicity. Zinc can also reduce the adverse effects of an excess of copper. Calcium can help in cases of aluminium overload, selenium in mercury toxicity. Other nutrients can help too. We haven't the space here to go into details. What is important is to warn you of the consequences of toxic minerals to your health and energy, encourage you to do the tests and then to work on whatever the results indicate should be done to improve the situation.

Mercury Amalgams

One of the most toxic metals that humans ingest is mercury. It is also one currently receiving a lot of attention. Many people are becoming aware of the situation and wondering about the advisability of having their amalgams removed and replaced with less toxic fillings. For this reason and since it is implicated as a possible contributing factor in CFS, it is considered here in some detail.

Not so long ago, it was considered normal to treat haemorrhoids with mercury-based suppositories. That has now been recognised as a dangerous practice. More recently, it was routine to plug dental cavities with a mercury amalgam. It seems we learn slowly, but gradually dentists are realising this is a dangerous practice. Far from being inert, the mercury in fillings leaks out into the mouth, encouraged by hot foods, active chewing and vigorous brushing. Since this mercury is in the mouth and the saliva, it is swallowed, absorbed and travels throughout the body.

Mercury causes a variety of symptoms and gave rise to the Mad Hatter's behaviour in *Alice in Wonderland*. For our purpose, it is interesting to note a report that of 705 people suffering from fatigue, 603 reported a significant increase in energy, many of them finding that their energy returned to normal, after removal of their mercury amalgams. Recall how important the immune system is in CFS (diagram). We know that mercury reduces the activity of the immune system. It also combines with oxygen in the red cells so that oxygen cannot be released when needed and this too is clearly an important contributing factor to CFS.

Whether or not you should have your amalgams removed is a personal decision. Some people have benefited enormously from doing this, but it is costly and

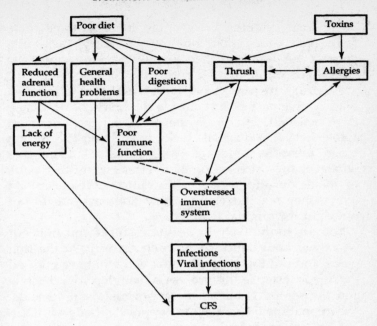

some people feel they have had little benefit from the expense and inconvenience. There is also the danger of mercury exposure as the amalgam is being removed. If the procedure is carried out with full and proper care, the risk is negligible but if you have CFS, a mouth full of amalgam fillings and do decide to have them out, then check out your dentist and the procedure s/he proposes to use very carefully. Whatever you do, do not have mercury amalgams put into your mouth ever again.

Drugs and Medication

All medical drugs have side-effects, no matter what you have been told to the contrary. I have listened to many patients who were assured that the drug they were pre-scribed was perfectly safe and when they complained of subsequent symptoms, were told it might have come from their medication, but not to worry, there was another medication that they could have to reduce the side-effects of the first.

All drugs are foreign substances, designed to interfere with or change a process inside the body. At best, they have beneficial effects on the problem with minimum side-effects. If you are less lucky, in addition to lowering blood pressure, reducing pain and inflammation, or whatever they also act on or interfere with other parts of the body and result in unwanted side-effects. At worst, they may cover up your symptoms but do not put right the original fault.

You are more likely to be successful if you find out why your body failed to function correctly in the first place, and put this right. By now you will have realised that the first step in this process is changing your lifestyle and the second is taking the appropriate supplements. Nutritional medicine aims to supply the body with the nutrients it needs, substances that are required by the body on a daily basis, are beneficial and do no harm even if provided at several times the required level. That is not to say that a huge excess of some nutrients is wise, any more than it is wise to drink many times the amount of water you need. But any possible adverse side-effects are usually minimal, even if you wildly overdose, and usually diminish with cessation of dosage.

The next step is to use herbal or homeopathic remedies which are in general sympathetic to the body and have only good side-effects. Nutrients will help to prevent fatigue. Drug medicines, on the other hand, will often contribute to it. As often as not, you can find a nutritional, herbal or homeopathic remedy that will solve the problem and thus allow you to avoid the chemical drugs.

Many drugs have fatigue as a side-effect; antihistamines are a common example. The drugs we are particularly concerned with here are antibiotics. You have already discovered how readily antibiotics can lead to an overgrowth of *candida* or thrush in the vagina and digestive tract and contribute to systemic candidiasis, and we also know that people with CFS commonly have candidiasis. A common scenario may well be poor nutrition leading to poor immune function followed by a viral or bacterial infection for which you are given an antibiotic. This antibiotic may then lead to candidiasis which becomes another confounding factor on your road to CFS.

Ideally, you should not use antibiotics. Certainly do not use them for a cold or the flu. As we discussed earlier (Chapter Seventeen), they will do nothing to help protect you from a virus yet are frequently taken at such times, when they do nothing positive whatsoever and only cause problems. Even when you have a bacterial infection, there is so much else you can do that you should find you very rarely need to take an antibiotic. The risk of developing candidiasis is too great to take without a great deal of thought.

Another common medication that can lead to candidiasis and to CFS is the contraceptive pill. There are alternatives and now, with AIDS a part of our lives and 'safe sex' so important, the emphasis is at last being taken off the contraceptive pill. Whatever you decide to do later, once your CFS is a thing of the past, give up the pill now.

Summary

- Have a hair sample sent for analysis.
- Have allergy testing done.
- Remove all toxins from your environment.
- Stop taking the contraceptive pill.

- Stop taking antibiotics and, if possible, stop taking any other medication, but check first with whoever prescribed this medication.
- Find alternative therapies for the treatment of any problem for which you care currently taking medication.
- Buy and start using a reverse osmosis water purifier.
- Find a source of organically-grown fruit, vegetables and grains, free-range eggs, etc.

References

Foundation for Toxic Free Dentistry compilation on 1569 Patients from Six References, *Bioprobe Newsletter*, March 1993.

Chapter Twenty-Seven

Treatment B – Internal Health

Your Digestive System

If anything you swallow, imbibe or otherwise consume is going to do you any good, your digestive system must be in good working order. We have said a lot about it already (Chapter Three), but it is now time to list and describe all the things you should do to make yours as healthy as possible.

There are many reasons why the digestive system is the important first step. We'll run through the reasons again, briefly. Firstly, it is the delivery system for all the nutrients needed by the rest of your body. If there are errors within the digestive tract that reduce or inhibit the absorption of dietary nutrients, you will be nutrient compromised even if your diet and your supplement programme are good. Secondly, if the wrong types of organisms are present in the system, you will be deprived of the ones that manufacture some of the important nutrients for you, such as vitamin K and several of the B group vitamins. Thirdly, if the biology and chemistry of the digestive tract are faulty you could have a number of toxic compounds generated there which, once absorbed into the bloodstream, could cause you a variety of adverse symptoms, including fatigue. Fourthly, if the breakdown of food is poor and the walls of the digestive tract are damaged, you could absorb partially-digested foods, which might then be recognised by your defence system as foreign and you could become allergic to them. Fifthly, part of the activity of your immune system starts and takes place here and if you are suffering from the consequences of viral problems you want your immune system to be as healthy as possible.

What To Do

Phase I
At this stage there is no problem with fasting. However tired you are, you already know that eating does not necessarily give you energy. Instead, this is a good time to give your digestive system a rest. It is also important to cleanse it. So ideally you should have only the things listed below for a few days, possibly a week or even ten days. Once any changes in your digestive system have occurred and settled down, you are ready to move on. If you are overweight, any loss in weight can only be beneficial. If you are underweight, you should move on to Phase II after three days.

1. Drink aloe vera juice. Find the purest you can. It should taste pleasant, perhaps as unusual as a glass of white wine the first time you taste it. It should not taste bitter or unpleasant. Keep in mind, however, that it is an acquired taste – but then again, so was wine when you first drank it.

There is often some confusion about aloe vera, some doctors or naturopaths telling patients it is a laxative and used for constipation; others that it is not, so an explanation here is appropriate.

When the whole leaf from the aloe vera plant is used to make a herbal extract, it is indeed an irritant to the digestive tract and as such is used as a laxative or purgative. Although its action is not violent, it may cause some griping. We are not interested in that action here and to understand what you do want, some knowledge is required of the leaf.

There are over two hundred types of aloe some of which are more beneficial and healing than others. It is a succulent (as are cacti). Its leaf is long, from a few inches to one or two feet long or more, and relatively flat, usually up to about an inch or two thick. At the base it can be several inches wide, tapering to a point at the end furthest from the plant. Along the two edges of the leaf there are spikes. These are the tips of spines that run through the leaf, inside, down to the base. Inside the skin and surrounding the spines is a clear jelly.

When you make a herbal extract using the whole leaf, you get the laxative and griping effect. When you use only the clear jelly from the centre you get the healing benefit of the plant without the laxative effect. This is the effect you want.

Now it is obviously easier, since no two leaves are the same shape and size, and the manufacturers supplying the juice want to extract all of the precious jelly they can, to use a mechanical processing method that extracts all the jelly and not too much of the external leaf. Ideally, however, you want a juice made from jelly that has been cleanly separated from the skin and spines and contains *none* of the outer leaf. It is not always easy to find out how a particular type of juice has been prepared, but the taste and smell can be a guide. If your aloe vera juice tastes bitter, is green or cloudy, it is not what you want. It may be cheap (and probably is), but it is not going to provide nearly as much healing benefit as a pleasant-tasting juice and it may be sufficiently cathartic to aggravate your problems – but make sure that a pleasant taste is not the result of the addition of sugar or other unwanted additives.

The great advantage of aloe vera from our point of view is that it is healing. I have had patients with ulcers, colitis, hiatus hernias and all sorts of digestive pains find rapid, prolonged and sustained relief from drinking about 50 ml or two fluid ounces of aloe vera juice three or four times a day. One man had had stomach ulcers for thirteen years and was eventually in such pain that he slept sitting up and would walk around the house at intervals all through the night. During the day he'd often be seen clutching his stomach in pain and he was always wary of what he ate. Within six weeks of starting to drink aloe vera juice regularly, in combination with slippery elm powder which we will discuss in a minute, he was pain-free. Another man, who had occasional bouts of pain from a suspected ulcer, starting in the early evening and worsening progressively till they reached an unbearable climax in the early hours of the morning, was saved many trips to hospital by additional doses of aloe vera juice. The moment the pain started, he started to sip it, very slowly and in tiny amounts but almost continuously. To my knowledge, he has had no more bad attacks, and only a few mild ones since he started this treatment

You may not have such a severe problem, but you will certainly have some damage to the intestinal wall. Processed foods, tea, coffee, alcohol, stress, medications, food additives – the list of the things that can damage the walls of the digestive tract is endless and we have already seen how allergies can result, as well as malabsorption of essential nutrients and other problems. Further, the mould form of *candida albicans* can have a devastating effect on the walls of the intestinal tract, doing considerable damage – think of how mould growing on a loaf of bread can damage the crust.

You can safely assume that if you have any digestive problems whatsoever, there is some damage to the mucosal lining, the walls of the intestinal tract, and the delicate hair like microvilli that line the intestines and give it the appearance of an internal crew cut. Even if you have no overt symptoms, there is likely to be some damage at the microscopic and local level, and I have had hundreds of patients who have benefited from drinking aloe vera juice daily. With CFS, it is an essential part of your treatment.

2. Eat slippery elm powder. One teaspoon night and morning is often sufficient. Put a small amount in water and watch what happens. It develops into a somewhat glutinous, mucilaginous liquid or paste that sticks to surfaces. When you swallow it, it leaves a fine covering along the walls lining your digestive tract, like putting on an internal bandage. This protects any damaged or ulcerous area and diminishes the amount of new damage that can be done. Obviously this layer is not stable and, with time, is dispersed through to the colon. Here it acts as a non-digestible carbohydrate (see Chapter Three) and helps to prevent constipation. Because it does not remain in one place, it is necessary to keep taking it two or three times a day.

In old days, it was made into a drink with warm milk and taken before bed, much as you might now make a Milo, Ovaltine or hot chocolate drink. If you do not like it as a drink, and I find some patients do but others definitely do not, then an easy way to take it is to mash it into a small banana. This almost entirely masks both the taste and texture and is an easy way of getting it down.

If you have a bout of severe pain from an ulcer, a hiatus hernia or something you simply call 'heartburn', then take a teaspoonful of this and the pain relief can be fast and total. Otherwise, have a teaspoon three times a day during this part of the treatment.

Slippery elm protects and aloe vera heals. In combination the two are an essential start to your treatment programme.

3. We have seen that getting the right organisms in the digestive tract is essential. The wrong ones do you a lot of harm and deprive you of a lot of nutrients. It is impossible for you to be totally healthy until this intestinal microflora is corrected.

Many people think that eating yoghurt is sufficient to accomplish this and that it will give them all the good organisms they need, but unfortunately this is not true. The important organism that you want is *lactobacillus acidophilus*, the acid-loving lacto (milk) bacillus. It is not surprising that this gives yoghurt its sharp, 'acidic' flavour. Unfortunately, although people like to think they are eating yoghurt and improving their health, they also, for the most part, like sweet things and not the acidity of acidophilus yoghurt. Many of the commercial yoghurts therefore contain *lactobacillus bulgaricus* and *streptococcus thermophillus*. These make pleasant-tasting yoghurts but the organisms can come to grief in the acid environment of the stomach and may not survive to reach the small intestine where you want them.

The above applies to the 'natural' or plain yoghurts. Most yoghurts will do you very little good at all in terms of re-inoculating your digestive tract since the ones that are the most popular are the flavoured yoghurts. These are coloured and flavoured to give the impression of being full of fruit, and are sweetened to please the palate and override any taste of real yoghurt. They are better described as pleasant 'custards' rather than real yoghurts. The plain yoghurts are very much better than the flavoured ones. However, many of the 'natural' yoghurts taste relatively sweet and have little or no *lactobacillus acidophilus*, the organism that you want. Even the 'natural' and plain yoghurts with a good acid bite to them probably have far too few organisms to make a major impact on your disturbed digestive tract.

Yoghurts can have a wide variety of organisms in them and this is fine when your are healthy and not suffering from candidiasis. What you want now is the pure form of *lactobacillus acidophilus*. It can be obtained in tablet form although many tablets, when analysed, do not have nearly as many viable organisms in them as are listed on the label. In fact they may contain, according to some analyses of different brands of tablets, less than ten per cent of what is claimed on the label. It is important that they come from a reputable company and have been correctly stored – many of them need to be kept refrigerated at all times.

Acidophilus can also be obtained in powdered form; this too should be kept in the refrigerator. Some people recommend the powdered form; others prefer a time-release tablet that is designed to see the organisms safely through the stomach and into the intestines where they are wanted. You would be wise to get some good advice as to the brand and type of supplement you take. You may also benefit from taking some bifidus as well as the acidophilus. This also comes in powdered form and needs to be kept refrigerated.

4. Most people are constipated. You are unless you normally have at least three large and bulky motions a day. At this time of repairing your digestive system, preparatory to a detox programme, it is particularly important that you clear out all the rubbish. To do this you need a gentle fibre, one that will move things along naturally.

Do not resort to laxatives, thinking that a thorough

cleanout is better than a gentle one. Laxatives simply
irritate the walls of the intestines, leaving them exhausted after each evacuation and so even less likely to perform for you next time. Eventually, if you continue to
use laxatives, you can become laxative-dependent, your
colon refusing to work on its own.

It is the gentle effect of fibre, swelling up and encouraging the intestinal walls into action, that you want.
Slippery elm will assist in this but you will need more.
Psyllium hulls, ground fine, are good. Linseeds are excellent and can be eaten whole or ground, but if you grind
them you should only do as much as you are going to
eat immediately as the precious unsaturated fatty acids
in the linseeds can go rancid very quickly. Other fibres
are excellent, including corn bran, oat bran, soy fibre,
apple fibre and pectin and a variety of others.

Not only should you be moving things along, you also
want substances that will absorb many of the toxins and
carry them along too. Most of these plant fibres, or non-
digestible carbohydrates, will do this. They will absorb,
for instance, the toxins from the dead *candida* cells and
so help to eliminate them from your intestines.

5. If you have reason to suspect that you have thrush or
have the *candida* organisms in the digestive tract, you
should take a few drops of propolis tincture three times
a day to assist in the process of getting rid of them.
Propolis is an anti-fungal and is made for and used by
bees for this purpose.

6. Drink lots of water. Two to three litres a day is a good
idea. This can be in the form of purified water, mineral
water, herbal teas, dandelion coffee or soups. Do not
include alcohol, tea or coffee. (You will not be drinking
these anyway during this fasting period.) They are
diuretic and so would increase your need for extra fluid.

Drinking plenty of fluid is important for a number of reasons. Most people drink too little water and this risks tissue dehydration. In the brain, this is thought to be a possible cause of structural shrinkage and poor memory and possibly a factor contributing to senility. The kidneys need an adequate amount of fluid for filtration and secretion of toxic wastes. Your immune cells, the ones that fight, engulf and destroy bacteria and so forth, need fluid to be able to move freely throughout your body and do their job. Finally, if your mucus membranes, such as your mouth, digestive tract, lungs and the genito–urinary area, are dry, it is much easier for viruses to enter and moulds to do damage than when they are moist.

7. If you decide you absolutely cannot go three days without food, have some boiled brown rice, but nothing else. If you have lost a lot of weight and are unacceptably thin then *do* include the brown rice in the programme from the start.

Summary

For the first three to ten days you will be taking the following:

- Aloe vera juice, at least 50 ml four times a day, more if you wish.
- Slippery elm powder, at least one teaspoon three times a day, more if you wish (mashed into half a banana if you need this to get the powder down).
- *Acidophilus* and *bifidus*, as recommended on the label, more if wished.
- A fibre supplement such as ground psyllium hulls, sufficient to have three large and soft motions a day.
- Propolis tincture, five drops three times a day.

- Purified water, two to three litres a day.
- Brown rice if you are underweight or feel you simply cannot fast on the above, as little as possible.

You will almost certainly have reactions to this programme as a lot of body changes will be occurring. You may feel a bit nauseous, you may get a headache, coated tongue, sore throat or produce extra mucus. You will, of course, feel hungry, but keep in mind that this fast is only going to last a few days. Find something pleasant to do to take your mind off your hunger pangs. Obviously this must be relaxing. Since you have CFS, your energy will be low anyway, and you should always take things easy when you are fasting. However, you may be able to organise pleasant surroundings, such as a beach with the ocean to watch or even swim in, or a country retreat. If you like music, opera, ballet or films, stock up with your favourites on disc or video. Plan to have someone give you a massage. Enjoy your favourite scents, have good friends around to chat with you or stock up on good books. There are many things you can do to make it an enjoyable time. This will help compensate for the fact that you are not eating. It will also lift your spirits and that is an important part of getting well again. If you simply fast but do nothing nice to compensate, you will possibly feel even more depressed and deprived than you do now.

If you have a severe reaction to this programme, it will be important to provide support for your liver. We'll consider that in the next chapter. You can, of course, do all this without supervision, since there is nothing inherently harmful in what you are doing – in fact, it is a highly beneficial programme. However, since some pretty major changes are going to be occurring in your body you might feel happier having someone who can give you advice or support and is experienced in this form of therapy. It is not essential, but it is something for you to think about.

Detoxification

We shall assume that you have completed Phase I for three to ten days or so. Not only have you started the process of repairing your digestive system and correcting some of the faults, you will also have started a detoxification programme. You will now be slimmer and leaner. You will feel 'cleaner'. You will also have noticed some changes. Your bowels should be working better, you may have been, or may still be, experiencing gas and wind and you may have noticed changes in the nature of your stools, changes in texture, colour, smell and frequency.

If you have a headache, it is almost certainly part of the detoxification. Other related symptoms include bad breath, a sour or unpleasant taste in the month, nausea, and a coated tongue. These symptoms are not a reason to abandon the programme. If you were totally healthy, in the sense that your digestive system was functioning correctly and well, and if you had no toxins stored away, the above programme would not cause you any problems and would not give you these symptoms. The symptoms are caused by your own system; the programme is the trigger that has started the beneficial changes.

It's a bit like spring cleaning. Just because it makes a mess, you do not blame the cleaning process and decide to stop what you are doing and stuff everything back into the cupboards. You recognise that the more rubbish there is to clear out, the more important it is that you get on and give the place a thorough clean. The same is true here. The worse your reactions to Phase I, the more important it is that you continue with the programme.

Phase II

After the first few days, possibly a week or so, your symptoms brought about by Phase I will settle down and then stop. You will be feeling better, lighter and healthier. It is now time to move on to Phase II. Do not be tempted to do this too soon. If you do, you may find that you will have to start all over again. It is much better to make a thorough job of the programme the first time around.

As you start Phase II, you can start eating a few selected foods. Ideally these should be brown rice and vegetables low in salicylates. The list includes artichokes, asparagus, beans, beetroot, broccoli, Brussels sprouts, cabbage, carrot, cauliflower, celery, chives, lettuce, peas, onions, parsley, pumpkin, radish, spinach, squash and turnips. Avoid all fruits and avoid aubergine, capsicum, cucumber, gherkins, potato, tomato and, of course, any foods to which you are allergic. Do not eat fruit or drink fruit juice at this stage. Drink black dandelion coffee or tea for your liver.

It is also important that you get some protein, but not protein to which you might be allergic. There are several reasons why you need protein at this time, although many practitioners may fail to make this point since it is not part of the conventional or traditional fast or cleansing programme. Without adequate protein intake there can be considerable loss of protein tissue from the digestive tract, the liver and your immune system just at the time when you need them to be at their healthiest and strongest. Obviously, it must be non-allergenic protein or you will be causing problems just at the time when you are trying to minimise them. For this reason, milk, egg or soy protein are not suitable since these foods are very common allergens. Gelatine is not appropriate either. Some of the cheaper protein powders you buy from health food shops and pharmacies are made largely of gelatine-like protein. This may indeed be pure protein, but it is protein with at least two of the essential amino acids (methionine and tryptophan) missing and for this reason is of no value to you in building up your own protein tissues. You will soon find out just how important methionine is in your detoxification programme. You do not want to consume a protein powder that will further reduce your relative methionine level. Find a protein powder based on or made from food to which you are not allergic. This is essential.

Ideally, you should try to find a source of partially hydrolysed (or predigested) protein consisting of di- or tripeptides. This is protein that has been broken down to such an extent that the 'imprint' of the original protein food is no longer there. In other words, your body can no longer recognise the source of the protein or detect that it is something foreign, and so does not initiate an allergic reaction to it. This will be particularly important if you are highly allergic. An excellent source of protein for this hydrolysis process is lactalbumin. Hydrolysed lactalbumin is well absorbed and well utilised by the body and has an amino acid pattern similar to human tissue. It should be less than 1200 daltons in size and you may find this marked on the container. Approximately 40 g of such a protein hydrolysate should be consumed three times a day.

You may be able to find this if you ask for the special protein foods that are given to highly reactive babies who cannot digest either milk or soy products. It can be expensive, but if you are allergic or react to other proteins (or if you fail to improve) then this may be a necessary component of your recovery programme. It is not a gourmet delight as pure protein has very little flavour, but it is non-reactive and it will prevent tissue breakdown (catabolism) which commonly occurs on cleansing programmes based simply on vegetables, juices or rice. A mixture of amino acids is a possible alternative if you cannot find the partially-hydrolysed protein but is far from satisfactory as such a mixture is expensive and only about ten per cent as effective.

If you are absolutely sure you are not allergic to milk, egg or soy products, you can use a protein powder based on these.

Summary

You will be eating:

- Protein powder, 40 g three times a day.
- Brown rice.
- Salycilate-free vegetables.
- And drinking black dandelion coffee and purified water.
- It is also a good idea to continue with the aloe vera juice, the propolis tincture and the acidophilus and bifidus.
- Continue with the slippery elm powder and psyllium hulls if you do not have three or four easy, soft and bulky motions a day.
- Do *not* add in any other new foods.

This programme will encourage further detoxification and symptoms of the beneficial changes that are being brought about. Remember though that, just as in Phase I, the symptoms will not necessarily be pleasant. Just welcome them as a sign that you are making progress. During this time it is possible you will begin to feel an improvement in your energy, though for some people this does not start until Phase III.

After a week on this programme, possibly two or three, the major part of the detoxification should have occurred. You will recognise this as a time when your symptoms settle back to normal and there are none of the cleansing signs listed earlier, and you will be feeling much better, though not necessarily full of energy yet. If you do not know whether it is time to proceed further, you might want to get some professional advice. Equally, since this is a healthy eating programme, there is no problem if you want to continue for a while. It is better to be thorough and complete each stage fully, rather than do a partial job. In the latter case, as in Phase I, you may at some stage in the future have to start all over again, so do not be tempted to rush things.

Supplements and Antioxidants for Phase II

Step 1. Activation. You will recall that many of the toxins you have absorbed over the years are fat-soluble and stored in your liver and fatty tissues. Phases I and II are designed to mobilise these toxins.

There is an important enzyme system, called cytochrome P450 that plays a vital role in dealing with these fat-soluble toxins by oxidising them into forms that are water-soluble and can be transported out of the body. The enzymes involved in this activation need a variety of coenzymes to function at their best. These include vitamins B2, B3 and B6 and the minerals iron, magnesium, manganese, molybdenum and zinc. As a result of these oxidising reactions, highly reactive oxygen free-radicals are produced that could, if not dealt with, cause the production of other very reactive and toxic substances. To avoid the build-up of free-radicals and so reduce this risk of an unwanted oxidation side-effect you need additional amounts of the anti-oxidant nutrients, vitamins A, C and E, beta-carotene, the flavonoids and selenium. Beta-carotene is a valuable immune potentiator, having both antiviral and antitumour activity. Silymarin is an excellent antioxidant herb to use at this time.

Step 2. Conjugation. The next step is to join these activated substances to small polar molecules. For this, you need cysteine, glucuronic acid, glutathione, glycine, methionine and sulphate. Some of these, such as glucuronic acid and glycine, your body can make for itself. Others, such as the amino acids cysteine and methionine, you cannot make, so they have to come from your diet or from supplements. You need vitamins B6, B9 (folic acid) and B12, and the minerals magnesium and selenium. You also need the sulphur-containing amino acids, methionine and cysteine.[1] If any of these substances are not available, further free-radical damage can occur, particularly in the liver. Fortunately, they are all commonly available as or in supplements with only one exception. In most countries you can buy selenium in the health food shops or nutritionally-oriented pharmacies. In Australia you cannot, for some reason that remains incomprehensible since it is an essential nutrient and helps to prevent heart disease and cancer; so you would be well advised to consult with your doctor and get it, if you can, on prescription.

The results you obtain from the process of Detoxification, consisting of Activation and Conjugation, will guide you as to your ongoing needs.

(a) If your body has all it needs for both steps 1 (Activation) and 2 (Conjugation) to go ahead rapidly, you will achieve a rapid detoxification with minimal side-effects. In a few days you will feel a noticeable difference: you will *feel* less toxic. Some patients do describe it as feeling 'clean', as if their system has had a real clear-out. They say they are more alert and more clear-headed; they lose any bad taste in their mouth, their breath improves, they don't get headaches or feel nauseous. Furthermore their general well-being and their energy improve.

(b) If both steps happen slowly, the detoxification process will take longer and there will be a milder form of those symptoms while it is going on. This suggests that your liver has already been over-stressed, probably by a variety of toxins. You can usually speed the process up by increasing your intake of the nutrients and substances mentioned for both steps.

(c) If the Conjugation step is faster than the Activation step, you will have the same experience as in (b) above.

(d) In the intermediate possibility, where the Activation step 1 is going rapidly and the Conjugation step 2 is going slowly, there will probably be considerable adverse symptoms. You may even decide that this 'healing crisis', or 'detox reaction' is so strong that the cure is worse than the problem. It isn't, not in the long run, but it will be much easier if you help the process along by supplementing with more of the Conjugation step substances. If you are having trouble finding them, look for remedies that are designed to help the liver. If you still feel bad after a few days on Phase II, go back to Phase I for three days and repeat the cycle.

During Phase II, in addition to the specific supplements already listed, your supplement programme should include a multivitamin and a multimineral tablet.

If you find you are getting additional gas and bloating or abdominal cramping, include a supplement containing hydrochloric acid and stomach digestive enzymes. This should be taken *with* the *end* of meals. This timing allows your own digestive acids to work on the first half of the meal and then the supplement takes over and finishes the job. Another digestive aid with pancreatic digestive enzymes may also be needed, and it too can be taken with the end of the meal. Continue to drink the aloe vera juice and take the slippery elm powder and the acidophilus mentioned for Phase I.

Your liver is intimately and intensely involved in this detoxification programme. Many of the detox enzymes occur in the liver, as do many of the reactions that occur in the Activation and Conjugation processes. Your liver will also have stored up a considerable quantity of the toxins, in a somewhat self-sacrificial protective process. For these reasons, it is important to support your liver, nutritionally and possibly with remedies as well. The nutrients you are already taken, as given above, play a major role in this. This includes nutrients such as methionine, the B group vitamins, vitamin C and many of the trace minerals.

There are other things you can do for your liver. One of these is to drink dandelion tea or coffee. Be sure, however, that it is not the instant variety that is sweetened with lactose. There is the chance that you may be milk or lactose sensitive and this could cause problems. Buy the dandelion root that has been roasted and ground. Simmer it gently for a while, strain and drink it as part of your fluid intake. There are also specific remedies for your liver, such as the homeopathic, Chelidonium.

If you are not allergic to soy, then lecithin granules will be valuable. They act as an emulsifying agent and are valuable in a variety of liver functions. They can be sprinkled on your vegetables, added to some other food you are eating, or washed down with a glass of water.

You may also find your joints and muscles are becoming stiff or painful. This could be due to acidic waste products or to inflammation brought about by allergens or toxins. Eating more vegetables, which contribute to the alkalinity of the body will help, so will drinking more water. The following combination is also helpful: mix one teaspoonful of sodium or potassium bicarbonate with one teaspoon of vitamin C powder, either a natural, plant-derived source or else sodium ascorbate, and take a supplement containing magnesium glycinate. Make this mixture up fresh each time you take it, since the bicarbonate can damage the vitamin C if they are mixed together for any length of time.

Although you have repeatedly been warned of the danger of oxygen free-radicals and the damage of oxidation to your tissues unless they are protected by antioxidants, it is still important that your cells and tissues get sufficient oxygen. You need oxygen for the normal metabolic pathways to operate and for the detoxification to take place; it is just that you also need to have the antioxidants to protect your own tissues from oxidative damage. It may be that your cells are not getting sufficient oxygen or that they are using it sluggishly.

An important nutrient, in this regard, is coenzyme Q10. This helps the mitochondria, those cellular power-houses where nutrients are converted into energy, to function efficiently. Another important supplement is dimethyl glycine (or DMG) which not only improves oxygenation but also, as a methyl donor, helps the liver and provides two conjugating agents, the methyl groups and the glycine.

When you have a high level of toxins, it is probable that your immune system has been overloaded and over-stressed. If you have CFS, it is likely that you have had a recent history of frequent infections. For these reasons you may also want to help your immune system along. One way to do this, of course, is to stop the overload. That is why it is so important, particularly at this time, to make sure your foods have been organically grown and that you do not eat foods that have been processed with a variety of added chemicals. It is also important that you avoid environmental toxins as we have said in Chapter Twenty-six and any foods to which you may be allergic (Chapter Eighteen) or which may contain moulds or yeasts (Chapter Sixteen).

Vitamin C is very important for your immune system and you could benefit from taking a few thousand mg a day. Find a powdered form, preferably from plant sources such as acerola, rosehips, citrus fruits and so forth and take a teaspoonful two to six times a day. If you get diarrhoea from this, it is a sign that you cannot absorb it quite as rapidly as you are swallowing it so reduce the dose slightly. If you cannot find a plant form, choose either ascorbic acid or sodium ascorbate, do not use calcium ascorbate, and add a supplement with the bioflavonoid complex to work with the vitamin C.

Some people find that even when they follow the above procedure, they do not fully recover. If this happens to you it may be that, in your present state of CFS, you cannot obtain sufficient vitamin C by mouth to have an adequate impact on your immune system and that you would benefit enormously from intravenous vitamin C. You should discuss this with a practitioner that specialises in this treatment.

Beneficial herbs for your immune system include echinacea and red clover. They can be drunk as teas, particularly the latter, or taken as supplements.

General Diet

Phase III

Once you have improved the state of your digestive system and gone through the detoxification programme you are ready to expand your diet. Be sure, however, to continue to exclude all foods to which you are allergic and all foods that are fermented or have yeasts or moulds in them (see the list in Chapter Sixteen). Initially you should continue to avoid all the grains other than millet and rice, all dairy products in any form, eggs, soy, peanut, beef, potato and tomato as these are common allergens and may possibly be a problem for you even if they did not show up on the allergy testing. You should, of course, continue to avoid all processed foods and foods with colours, flavours, preservatives and other added chemicals.

Avoid sugar. Apart from all the other problems it can cause, sugar actually weakens your immune system. It does this by competing with vitamin C to enter cells and you already know that vitamin C is important for your immunity. Your immune cells, the white blood cells, contain as much as one hundred times as much vitamin C as other cells. Vitamin C is important for the function of these cells and you do not want to give them the chance to take up sugar instead.

Ideally, all the foods you do eat should be organically grown so that you avoid the intake of the various agricultural chemicals that would otherwise have been applied to them.

As your health improves, add in the other unprocessed foods listed above, such as the grains, unless you know you are allergic to them, but continue to avoid foods with any added chemicals or that have been processed. If any food seems to cause your problems, eliminate it from your diet.

Continue to drink dandelion coffee or tea and have at least two (and preferably three) litres of fluid a day. Remember, the water you drink and use in cooking should be filtered and have passed through a reverse osmosis membrane as discussed earlier.

Diet and Supplements for CFS

When we considered energy and nutrients in earlier sections, we covered the ways the different vitamins, minerals and other nutrient factors contributed to normal energy production in the body. Exactly the same pathways and the same considerations apply to someone with Chronic Fatigue Syndrome, but here they are even more important. It is simply that whilst providing these nutrient factors was sufficient to get the person lacking in energy back on their feet again, this is no longer sufficient in itself when you have CFS. For the treatment of CFS, you have had to go through the procedure outlined above.

Make sure you have a diet composed mainly of raw fresh fruits and raw and lightly-cooked fresh vegetables, preferably organically grown. Use whole grain products with a minimum of processing and incorporate low-fat proteins, especially fish. If your liver is functioning well and can handle them, beans (the dried variety such as red kidney beans, haricot beans and the various lentils and split peas) provide useful protein. However, bear in mind that they contain an enzyme inhibitor and can depress your intestinal protein digestion if your enzyme production is inadequate. You will soon know. If you feel the slightest indigestion after eating these foods or if your abdomen is bloated or you pass wind after eating them, you would be advised to give the legumes a miss. Raw seeds such as sunflower and sesame are good nutrient sources provided you chew them well.

You will almost certainly benefit from being on an anti-*candida* programme which means you will have to continue to avoid all the foods that contain yeast or moulds or have been fermented. You will also have had allergy checks done and should continue to avoid all your allergens. It is essential that you avoid these totally, at least for a few months, to give your body and particularly your immune system a chance to recover and normalise.

Eat small and frequent meals. This way you avoid the chance of hypoglycaemic slumps. You also give your digestive system the chance to digest small amounts of food at a time by not overloading it. Make sure you relax both while you eat and afterwards for an hour or two. Do not drink with meals as you want your stomach acids to be as concentrated as possible.

Summary

Phase I   Fast for three to ten days avoiding everything except that which will heal your digestive system – slippery elm powder, aloe vera juice etc, as listed.

Phase II   Include brown rice, selected vegetables that are low in salicylates and non-allergenic protein; and do this for up to three weeks, until your symptoms have settled. Take the supplements indicated to help (a) Activation and (b) Conjugation.

Take the general supplement programme and add other specific nutrients as indicated.

Phase III   Expand your diet to include all 'good' foods that are not either on the mould yeast list or an allergen. Continue to avoid all junk and processed foods.

---

[1] For details on Activation and Conjugation, I am indebted to discussions with M. Curly, Health World, Austrlia.

Chapter Twenty-Eight

Treatment C – Associated Health Problems

If you have followed the treatment programme so far, you are well on the way to developing a lifestyle that will get you back to full and vibrant health. By now, you should have done the following:

- Sent a hair sample off for analysis.
- Had allergy testing done.
- Eliminated all the toxins you can from your environment.
- Fasted for three to ten days while cleansing and healing your digestive system – Phase I.
- Spent up to three weeks on a detox programme, eating brown rice, selected vegetables and non-allergenic protein and taken the appropriate supplements – Phase II, Activation and Conjugation plus immune support.
- Expanded your diet to include good foods but continued to omit moulds and yeasts, your allergens and all processed foods and those with any chemical additives.
- You've considered the possible need for
  (a) Stomach and pancreatic digestive enzymes.
  (b) Alkalising treatment for muscle and joint pains.

(c) Improving cellular oxygenation.

(d) Improving immune function.

In this section, we shall be covering other forms of therapy you should add to what has already been described. Some of this will refer you back to other parts of this book; some of it may sound repetitious. I can only assure you, after over twenty years in clinical practice, that repetition is very necessary. It is so easy to 'forget' the instructions you don't want to hear, or to underestimate the importance of each step along the way. Further, as mentioned above, if you know you have CFS you may have jumped straight to this section of the book, so you may have to be referred back to the appropriate parts of the previous three sections.

Firstly, for CFS, as for any other form of tiredness and energy loss, it is essential that you check for the possibility of any other health problem that could be contributing to your problem. Go back and consider the various chapters in Parts II and III.

Check back to the chapters on the way your thyroid and adrenal glands function. If you have any reason to suspect that specific treatment is needed for either of these glandular systems, go ahead and include that in your programme (see Chapters Ten and Eleven). Reread the chapter on anaemia (Chapter Nine) and, if you think it is appropriate, take a supplement containing iron, folic acid and vitamin B12. Many people with CFS have been helped by a monthly shot of B12. This is usually injected into the muscles of the buttocks and the effect lasts about a month unless you consume large quantities of alcohol.

Do you suffer from stress? Do you feel overwhelmed by what you have to do and unable to cope? If so go back to Chapter Fourteen and consider what you can do to reduce or eliminate this stress. By now, in the programme, you will be taking most of the appropriate

supplements, but might want to consider whether you
need extra pantothenic acid (vitamin B5) or extra vitamin
C. The mental side is important. You do not have to feel
stressed. You are the one who decides whether or not
something will stress you. Now is the time to read the
appropriate books, go to the appropriate seminars or
find an appropriate psychotherapist. You can eliminate
the experience of stress from your life if you know how
to deal with it.

You may also have to talk with your family, friends,
colleagues or whoever is involved with your life, and
arrange a period of 'time-out' so you can rest and
recover. They need to be told that this is not going to be
another holiday or a break, after which you will return
to your normal life only to find you are feeling no better.
Let them know that you are starting, or have started,
on a structured programme that will lead you back to
improved energy and health and that time-out to follow
this programme is essential for your health and well-
being.

Do you have hypoglycaemia? If so, pay attention to
the instructions given in Chapter Fifteen. In addition
to what you are already doing, which will be of enormous help, you may still need to eat small meals at
frequent intervals, rather than two or three main meals
in the day. It will be vital to avoid all yeasts and moulds,
all your allergens and all sugars, possibly even fruit and
fruit juices as well. I know we have already covered this,
but many people allow a few slips or errors to creep in
to their programme. If you have hypoglycaemia, it is
essential that you do not allow allergens, moulds or
sugars to slip in to your diet.

We have considered thrush or candidiasis in Chapter
Sixteen. Now would be a good time to go back to that,
read it again, and make sure that you incorporate into
your treatment programme all the suggestions given

there, in addition to the programme provided so far in this section. It is vital that you follow the full treatment process for candidiasis (Chapter Sixteen). You may not know whether or not candidiasis is part of your problem. However, it is so common today and particularly among those with symptoms of CFS that you would be foolish to try to go ahead without doing this.

You will recall the diets and supplements that were recommended for thrush. We also spoke of the need for special bedding and ensuring there were as few dust surfaces as possible, that shelves were closed behind glass doors, and so forth. Follow these instructions as far as is convenient, unless you have respiratory symptoms in which case you should follow them completely. If you have CFS, as opposed to simple candidiasis, you may have to make even more extensive changes. You may have to pull up all the carpets and have polished or tiled floors instead. Is your house damp? Could that situation be improved? Some houses are just inherently damp. If you rent, you may consider moving. If you own, the decision is obviously a bigger one, yet a move may be necessary if you are to recover your full health and energy. If you cannot move, do all you can to reduce damp throughout the house and make sure your room is the least damp. You may need to introduce ventilation to get a flow of fresh air,

If you have any reason to suspect you have acquired a parasite, been infected with a variety of unwanted intestinal organisms, or have worms, see someone who can do the appropriate tests for you. If you have been away on holiday, or in the tropics, you may have picked up something that could hold back your recovery. If you suspect any of these, a stool test and others as appropriate should be considered. Your doctor will be able to advise you on this.

Your immune system is important and we have

already discussed it. You will find that the programme you are now on, as a result of Phases I to III, is of inestimable value to your immune system and you will have much greater resistance to infections in future. In addition to the nutrients discussed, the herbs echinacea and red clover help to boost the immune system, as do the mushrooms reishi and shitake. These are sometimes combined and sold as Re-Shi-Gen.

Mention has been made in earlier chapters of your liver and its importance. It plays so many vital roles, from dealing with and breaking down toxins to its various roles in iron and vitamin metabolism. It is essential for the normal metabolism of fat and for eliminating cholesterol and thus benefiting your heart. It is a vital part of your digestive system, handling and altering the nutrients you have absorbed so that you can extract benefit from them. If you are unwell, you may say you are feeling 'liverish'.

Your liver is almost certainly struggling if you have CFS. To assist it, make sure you take a full spectrum of all the B group vitamins and the trace minerals, particularly selenium, zinc, manganese and copper. The amino acids methionine and cysteine, obtained from eggs or in supplement form, are important and so is lecithin, which can be used either as a food in granule form or as a supplement in tablet or capsule form. Dandelion is an excellent herb for the liver and can be obtained as a coffee or tea. In health food shops you will find a variety of products specifically aimed at supporting your liver, containing the above and other beneficial ingredients.

If you have any reason to suspect a specific health problem, this should be checked for and dealt with. However, let's put that into perspective. If you have ever tried to clear a large and very overgrown garden you will know that there is little point in grabbing all the weeds from the top and hauling out as much as you can. If you keep doing that you may be pulling of a lot of different chunks of the same weed. The best way is to find the major root, pull this out, taking the entire plant with you, then look to see what is left and work on that in a similar fashion.

It is similar with CFS and many of your other health symptoms. You may indeed have eczema, you may have asthma and you may get hay fever from time to time. Yet the solution may not be to go to a doctor to get a broncho-dilator for the asthma, an antihistamine for the hay fever and cortisone cream for the eczema. By going back to the root, almost certainly your allergies, and any problems with your digestive and immune systems, and dealing with them, you may be able to resolve all three problems. When you do that, you may find that all you have left is an occasional, mild form of asthma and when you then go back to Chapter Twenty and are reminded that you might be needing extra vitamin D, calcium and magnesium and add them to your programme, the asthma goes entirely.

There is a bit of a chicken-and-the-egg situation here. The asthma can be contributing to the exhaustion, and the exhaustion and resultant stress can be causing the asthma. If you work in the structured way that is recommended in this Section, you should be able to solve all the problems. In addition, no matter whether your heart contributed to your fatigue, or your fatigue stressed your heart, both problems now exist and, since you presumably want to get as healthy as you can as fast as you can, you would be well advised to work from both ends, from the fatigue angle and on the heart problem or any other health problem, at the same time,

If you are overweight you may already find, following the few days of fasting and three weeks or more of rice and vegetables, that you have begun to lose weight. If losing more weight is your goal, stay on this programme and let the weight continue to decrease. Even when you add in the greater variety of healthy foods, you may still continue to lose weight. After all, this programme allows you no sweets, chocolates, cakes, biscuits, fried food, ice-cream, soft drinks and so forth, and these are probably what was causing the weight gain in the first place.

Exercise

Exercise is an important part of the therapy. 'No' you may shout. 'How can I possibly exercise when I am exhausted?' We are not talking about running marathons or sprinting the length of a football field. We are talking about mild exercise. You already know that rest and sleep have not helped you. Undoubtedly you have tried that. If your CFS symptoms are severe, you have been spending a lot of the day in bed, or lying around the house. This has not helped. You have slept a lot and you have almost certainly not woken up feeling refreshed.

Mild exercise helps to improve oxygenation of the cells. It improves the blood circulation to the tissues, which in turn improves their nutrition and oxygenation and helps the normal lymphatic drainage of toxins. A good way to start your exercise programme is by walking. Do not overtax yourself. Now is not the time to set records. Be content to do just a little bit each day, a little bit more than you have been doing, and to do it gently and without strain. You will not benefit by making a heroic effort to walk until you drop. Instead, go for a short walk each day and increase the length and duration gradually, as your detoxification and nutrition programs improve and your symptoms diminish. Make sure you are wearing really comfortable shoes with plenty of padding.

Swimming is another useful form of exercise, provided you can find clean water to swim in, as it does not jar the joints in the way walking may do. Swim in the ocean where there is a minimum pollutant level and avoid chlorinated pools as chlorine is a strong oxidising agent and will work against your detox programme.

Sleep

Many people who experience fatigue have simply been overdoing things or burning the candle at both ends. They know it, as do the people around them, and if they go to bed early for a couple of nights and get some extra sleep, they will bounce back, full of energy. If you are experiencing CFS you have almost certainly tried that already. You have slept. You may even have been sleeping ten to fourteen hours a day, but finding little benefit, often waking unrefreshed and almost as tired as when you went to sleep. Your muscles may still be tense and tight. It may be that your sleep has been shallow, disturbed by many small noises. You may have spent a restless night, remaining unconscious yet restless and with many dreams.

This can be caused or aggravated by a number of factors, including coffee, alcohol and a deficiency of magnesium or calcium. It can also come about if you have been doing no exercise and are aerobically unfit. That is one of the reasons you have been told to do some exercise, even if it is only enough to induce gentle aerobic activity. You may not be able to run a marathon but at least you will sleep better as a result.

You will sleep better if the environment is quiet. Normally, when you do not have CFS, when you are really tired you can fall asleep anywhere, no matter what the noise level, and sleep soundly until you are refreshed. When you have CFS this is more difficult and it is important to find as quiet a place as possible to sleep.

Obviously you will sleep less well and less deeply if

your mind is running round in circles. This is one of the reasons why you need to work on reducing your stress response to what is going on around you. Learning to meditate and relax is helpful, and you might benefit from the use of some audio tapes that have been designed to assist this.

Muscle and joint pains can disturb your sleep. Many joint and muscle inflammations, such as rheumatism and arthritis, are caused by allergies so these problems will often improve when you follow an allergen-free regime. Taking a combination of calcium, magnesium, manganese, zinc, copper and silica will also help the joints, particularly if the supplement contains vitamin A and D to assist with the absorption of calcium and the transport of zinc. You may also need stomach acid and enzymes to assist in the mineral absorption. If you find your legs twitch, try taking some extra vitamin E or the omega-3 fatty acids from fish. The best source is deep-sea fish, rather than salmon that swim in rivers and estuaries since these tend to be more polluted than the deep ocean. Do not use cod-liver oil or halibut-liver oil for this purpose, or you will get too much vitamin A and D before your intake of the fatty acids is sufficient to be beneficial.

Remember, if you are allergic to dust or dust mites, you will need the special bedding that helps reduce your exposure to these factors while you are in bed. Many people find that they feel worse in the morning simply because, as they are waking up, they move around in the bed and stir up both the dust and the mites and then, inevitably, breathe in the combination and react to it.

Oxygen

Oxygen, as you will have realised by now, is a mixed blessing. If you are exposed to either oxygen or oxidising agents and are deficient in antioxidants, you will suffer from oxidative and free-radical damage. However, if you are taking the full spectrum of antioxidants, as you should be by this time, your health will improve even further if you increase the amount of oxygen available to the cells and with which they can convert the foods you have eaten into energy.

The first step towards this goal is proper breathing. Short and shallow breathing will not do. Breathe slowly and regularly. Use the muscles of your diaphragm to pull long slow and big breaths of air into your lungs and down into the deepest part of them so that your full lung capacity is used. Let your abdomen stick out as you do this, you need all the internal space you can create. Then relax all these muscles and let all the air leave your lungs until they are as flat as they can be. Repeat the process. You will find this will make a huge difference to your energy level. If you are a singer, sing. This will increase the amount of air you draw in. Then let it all out as you sing your lungs out. You can make this diaphragm breathing even more effective if, for a while, you breathe through your mouth rather than your nose, keeping your lips pursed so that only a small amount of air can enter and leave and you have to draw it in actively. This gives your respiratory muscles something to work against.

At the cellular level there are a couple of nutrients that can increase the cells' uptake and utilisation of oxygen. Remember that oxygen has to enter the cells, travel across them and enter the mitochondria, the power-houses of the cell where the majority of the energy is produced.

One of these enzymes is coenzyme Q10, commonly referred to as CoQ10, which comes in tablet form and helps protect the mitochondria from free-radical oxidation and increases the efficiency with which your cells convert glucose into energy. Another is dimethyl glycine (or DMG), available as a liquid. DMG is a methyl donor, like methionine which we saw earlier helps with the Conjugation step of Phase II detoxification. This is particularly helpful for the liver which has a lot of work to do in the detoxification process.

Two minerals are important: magnesium and calcium. Magnesium is important for many reasons, mostly too technical to go into here. It is enough to say it is a coenzyme in many of the necessary and important oxidative reactions involved in converting fats and carbohydrates into energy. Calcium helps to prevent the build up of lactic acid that can cause muscle fatigue and pain.

Gentle, aerobic exercise, relaxed and deep sleep and thorough oxygenation of the cells will greatly help to reduce the muscle aches and pains that commonly occur as part of CFS.

Other Forms of Therapy

The treatment outlined in this section is the core of the treatment programme for CFS. There are many other things you can do to assist your recovery.

Chiropractic and Osteopathy

Chiropractic and osteopathic treatments will facilitate the process in many ways, although on their own they will not be sufficient. By improving your structure, nerve messages, blood and lymph flow, and stimulating your organs and all the other benefits these modalities can accomplish, they can assist in your recovery and add to the effectiveness of the rest of your programme.

Massage
Massage can help you relax. Abdominal massage can assist in the cleansing programme as it works on your intestine and colon and improves the peristaltic action. By releasing muscle tension and stimulating the flow of blood and lymph it can help in the removal of toxins from the tissues and the delivery of nutrients to the tissues.

Homeopathy
Low potency homeopathics are particularly useful in combination with this treatment. Use remedies, in appropriate sequence, that assist each step of the programme, first the digestion, then the detoxification, and combine the latter with remedies that support the liver's role in this. If you have specific health problems, use the homeopathics that help this aspect of your healing process.

Aromatherapy
As with homeopathy, you can pick the remedy, in this case the oils and the aromas, to support what you are doing in the treatment programme as it is outlined above.

Acupuncture
Acupuncture can help to stimulate energy flow, to improve the circulation and drainage and to energise the individual organs to make the maximum use of the nutrients and other treatments you are taking.

Others
Almost any other form of positive therapy that is in harmony with your body and the natural biological laws can be helpful. You must, of course, avoid the use of any toxins, whether they are chemical, such as medical or

other drugs, or physical, such as X-rays, electromagnetic fields so forth. Use only treatments that are non-invasive and have no known or recognisable adverse side-effects. You also want to avoid therapies that 'whip up' your energy. Their effect will be a shortlived and will be detrimental to the overall healing effect for which you are striving.

If you have put all this into practice, you should be well on the way not only to recovering your old energy back, but also to achieving a situation whereby you feel even better than you did before the problem started.

Chapter Twenty-Nine

Treatment D – Mental Changes

There is one final but major aspect of therapy for CFS and that involves the mental and emotional aspects of the situation and the treatment. Your mood, what you are saying to yourself, your expectations and assumptions, your attitude to the treatment, all these have an enormous bearing on your recovery potential and rate.

If you are depressed, if you are telling yourself it is hopeless, you are exhausted and have no energy for anything, that it's been like this for ages and there is no way out, you will hold back your recovery. Equally, if you view the steps along the way, the steps outlined in the earlier part of Part IV, as being inconvenient, difficult and more trouble than they're worth, then you probably won't stick to them and, even if you do, you will not put your heart and soul into the therapy. As a result, it will be less well done and less effective.

This is important for three reasons. It affects the way it makes you feel mentally. It affects your actions and commitment to the treatment. Thirdly, the way you think actually changes your cellular chemistry.

Your Thoughts and Your Cells

If you think about something of which you are afraid, you can actually change the amount of adrenalin coursing through your body. If you are depressed or grief-stricken, the number of your white cells decreases. This has been shown quite clearly by studies of elderly couples after one of the partners has died. You need those important white cells. They are part of your immune system and you have learnt how vital it is for that to be functioning to its maximum potential.

The placebo effect is so well recognised that it hardly needs discussion. We all know that if you are given a tablet and expect it to work, it probably will, even if it is only a dummy sugar-coated pill. It is impossible to get a valid picture of the benefit of a new drug simply by giving it to patients and waiting to find out what happens, without giving half the group a placebo so that the effect of positive assumption of benefit can be equalled out and the real effect of the drug ascertained. What many people fail to recognise, however, is that this means that when you feel positive and powerful you can assist your own healing, at any time, with or without a tablet. In the same way, when you feel positive about the treatment for your fatigue, the therapy will be that much more successful.

Your Thoughts and the Therapy

The treatments described in this book will work. They have worked for others. They will work for you. They have worked for thousands of people suffering from CFS and treated by a large number of different practitioners. To give yourself the best possible chance of being one of that number, it is important that you take this confidence on board yourself and that you enter the programme willingly.

I have watched patients who started on this or any other programme thinking of all the problems it could present, of the difficulties it could make in their social life, of their unwillingness to forgo their foods of choice, the processed and convenient foods they had come to love and that probably contributed to the problem in the first place. They focused on their dislike of taking tablets and their (misplaced) belief that they are not needed. They struggled to stick to the protocol, they complained it didn't work and, in some instances, came back some months or even a year or two later, sufficiently desperate that they were now willing to get started.

I have watched others take the more positive approach. They decided it was worth it. They recognised that a week or so on the cleansing and repair of the digestive tract, followed by one to three weeks on vegetables, brown rice and non-allergenic protein would only take a month or so out of their lives, a month during which, if they continued as they were, they would go on feeling exhausted. They recognised that if they wanted their health to change, they themselves must make some changes. They recognised that modern drug medicine has no drug that will solve their problem, that there is no form of surgery that could improve their energy and that they must look to a more rational solution.

I have seen people embrace this treatment programme so enthusiastically that they got excited about the changes that were going on in their body. The more they had cleansing reactions, the more thrilled they were that they were making progress. I recall one woman who boasted to me at each visit about the new and interesting ways she had found of preparing and serving the selected vegetables and rice. I recall a man who, after suffer-

ing from fatigue for thirteen years and finally collapsing
into CFS after treatment with prednisone for a skin rash,
was so excited by the fact that someone could finally
make sense of all his seemingly confusing symptoms
that he kept swearing he would stick exactly to *whatever*
he was told to do. He did, and the results were dramatic,
an immediate gradual improvement in energy followed
by a rapid recovery. I can think of many who have said
they were feeling so good on this programme that they
didn't want to change, they didn't want to add in more
foods, they didn't want to risk anything that would
reduce their growing feeling of well-being and energy.

The attitude you choose to take to this is just that,
your choice. It's a case of 'the method works – if you
do'.

Your Thoughts and CFS

Your thoughts are particularly powerful in relation to
CFS for a number of reasons.

Firstly, your thoughts and emotions have an immediate impact on your digestive system. When you are
frightened, angry, tense or experiencing some other
negative emotion, it is common to find that your mouth
goes dry, the saliva flow slows, and you find it difficult
to swallow food. These are the obvious changes. Similar
changes are occurring throughout your digestive tract, as
we saw earlier (Chapter Three). These negative emotions
stop the flow of that important stomach acid, they reduce
the output of digestive enzymes and they slow down
the peristaltic action that propels the food along. Your
thoughts affect your digestive system and you now
know how vital it is for your recovery from CFS that
this digestive system functions at its best. Negative
emotions will interfere with this.

Secondly, your thoughts and emotions affect your

immune system. Mention has been made of the reduction in the number of white cells that occurs when people are depressed or grieving. There are numerous examples of people who, when depressed or afraid, become more susceptible to infections and other health problems. You already know how important a healthy immune system is going to be to your recovery from CFS.

Thirdly, your thoughts will affect whether or not you stick to the programme. As you have seen, the programme demands discipline and some significant changes in your lifestyle. You do this on will-power, but not on will-power alone. If you try to, you will be setting up an internal battle, telling yourself you want your old lifestyle but that you can't have it while relying on your will-power to dominate your wants. That may work for a little while, but you cannot expect your will-power to beat the temptations all the time. The temptations you are fighting are like the North Sea pressing on the dams of Holland. They are relentless, they are there all the time, they will not let you rest or relax for a minute. You just need one moment of weakness, one moment when your defences are down and you will find yourself eating or drinking something you shouldn't, you will skip your tablets or load in the toxins. When you do this, you can set your progress back by days, even weeks.

The way to avoid this is not to tell yourself you still want what you cannot have and rely on will-power to fight the desire, but to embrace the new ways, recognising them as holding the seeds of the new, healthy and energetic you. Tell yourself you do want to give up the old junk foods, you do want to eat rice and vegetables, you don't want to be toxin-laden and tired, you do want to feel fresh and energetic. Above all, tell yourself you don't want what the old ways did to you.

Fourthly, whatever your state of health or level of

energy, you can feel better when you put a positive mental attitude into it than when you apply a negative one. If you think it will be a good day, it will be; you will notice the good things and, in many subtle ways, you will make good things happen. If you think it will be a bad day, it will; you will notice the bad things and again, in many subtle ways, you will make bad things happen. While your health and your energy are down, it is all the more important to change what you can, if you choose so to do – namely, your mental attitude.

Many books have been written on this, including four of my own, at least three of which are pertinent to CFS.[1] Read them, and books by other authors. Play tapes of affirmations and positive ideas. You may not have the energy to go to seminars, but there is a wealth of material around that you can have at home and work with, without expending too much energy.

Your Thoughts and Your Energy

There is one major thought that you should change that is also an essential part of the physical changes you worked with earlier. It is vital that you stop saying to yourself that you are tired and so must rest. It is essential that you break this association. The more you rest, the more unfit you become. By reducing your physical activity, you reduce your fitness and the oxygenation of your blood. It is essential that you avoid this hypoxia, this lack of oxygen. As you have read, you need the oxygen in your bloodstream to be available for the cells so they can burn up the food you have eaten and convert it into energy. You need to exercise, however gently.

A more useful and appropriate thought would be to think that you are tired, and tire easily, because you have not been doing enough (gentle) exercise to keep fit and have the energy you want. We spoke of exercise earlier, and I repeat, it should not be excessive. However, it is important, not only that you do gentle exercise, but that you start to associate the thought of being tired with not having done *enough* exercise, rather than with the thought that you must have been doing too much.

Your Thoughts and Control

At this stage you may not feel you have much control over your body. After all, every time you ask it to do something it refuses. You are too tired and, though the spirit may be willing, the flesh is weak. However, even at this stage, you do have control over your thoughts. This means that your therapy can start here. You can start with positive affirmations. It takes no energy to make them. You have to think something; it might as well be a positive thought as a negative one. It takes no energy to listen, so listen to tapes that encourage you along the lines of positive thinking. Listen to tapes that inspire you to move forward rather than remain where you are. It takes very little energy to read, although for some people their CFS is so severe that reading for any length of time is difficult, even holding a book may be too tiring. However, whenever you do read, make sure it is something positive that will help you take constructive steps forward. This is no time for reading for light enjoyment, for escapism, or to pass the time. Read books that will help you become healthier and be willing to take the (mental) exercise they require. If reading is definitely too difficult, ask someone to read to you. They can read a small section of a book on the way your mind can help you improve your health and then leave you to digest what has been read.

Your Thoughts and the Benefits of CFS

'Benefits?' you say. 'There are no benefits in having CFS.' Think about it. Do this in private, no one need know what you are thinking. What are some of the benefits of having CFS? Does it mean you do not have to face some of the challenges at work any more? Does it mean you no longer have to do jobs you hate to do? Is it a relief to find that people have fewer expectations of you than they had in the past? Perhaps you are getting more attention from family and friends. Perhaps the family expected you to do everything for them, you hadn't the heart to let them down, yet you now appreciate having a reason to lay down that burden. Perhaps people are showing more care and concern for you than they did when you were well, energetic and someone *they* could rely on. Perhaps a lover is not leaving you, now that you need them. Perhaps you were not keeping up with new developments in your career, now you have a reason to move sideways, take early retirement or change to a less challenging job.

There is no implicit blame or fault in any of this. Your unconscious mind is very clever at meeting your needs in the safest way possible (see *Choosing Health Intentionally*[1]) and it is often a lot safer to be sick and get sympathy and comfort than to come right out and ask someone how much they love or care about you. Don't shout. I can hear the protests from here, even as I write. Be willing to face your innermost thoughts. There is no harm in having them. The harm occurs when you continue to use CFS to get the results you want. If you want to make changes in your life, try making them without needing to be ill. Then you will be able to embrace your recovery programme without your subconscious pulling you back.

None of this is to say that you have consciously

created your CFS – though keep in mind that it *is* you who has done all the things that led you to this point. It *is* you who chose what you ate and drank and your environment, who did or didn't take supplements, and so forth. What is useful now is to realise that you can also make the positive choices needed for recovery. You can use this time to reassess yourself and your life. You may want to find a practitioner, a counsellor, who can help you come to terms with your hopes and your fears, who can help you redesign your future. You may decide to do it on your own.

Whatever it takes, the future is yours to choose and design. The first step is to recover your physical health. This can be done with the methods described here. The next step is to maintain this health and this will mean redesigning your lifestyle to maintain your new-found health. The methods for doing this are also to be found in this book. The third step, and you can be doing it at the same time, is to redesign your life emotionally.

This may seem like a lot of changes to make. But Chronic Fatigue Syndrome is a *major* health problem. It threatens the very basis of your life. It threatens your energy, your ability to use your body. It threatens your ability to function in the world, to do what you need to do not only for survival, but to have fun and to achieve your goals. Dealing with it is going to involve major action and major changes.

You now know how to do it. The rest is up to you.

References

Xandria Williams, *Choosing Health Intentionally*, Simon and Schuster 1990 (Australia), Charles Letts & Co. Ltd 1992 (UK).
Xandria Williams, *Stress – recognise and resolve*, Charles Letts & Co. Ltd, 1993.
Xandria Williams, *Beating the Blues*, Cedar, 1995.

INDEX

abbreviations
ADP, adenosine di-phosphate
ATP, adenosine tri-phosphate
CFS, Chronic Fatigue
  Syndrome
CMV, Cytomegalovirus
DMG, dimethyl glycine
EBV, Epstein-Barr virus
EPA, eicosa-pentaenoic acid
GTF, Glucose Tolerance Factor
GTT, glucose tolerance test
HDL, High Density
  Lipoprotein
LDL, Low Density
  Lipoprotein
NLP, Neurolinguistic
  Programming
RDA, recommended daily
  allowance
TRH, Thyroid-Releasing
  Hormone
TSH, Thyroid-Stimulating
  Hormone
VLDL, Very Low Density
  Lipoprotein

XANDRIA WILLIAMS

Liver Detox Plan
The Revolutionary Way to Cleanse and Revive Your Body

This cleansing, reviving and rejuvenating *Liver Detox Plan* has simple and practical ideas to help you lose weight, and tackle the wide range of health problems caused by the challenge of daily life.

Your liver handles hundreds of different reactions and its health affects every single part of your body. It may be the silent cause behind almost any symptom or health problem you may have, and it can be in trouble, even before you find yourself feeling 'liverish' or jaded either in general, or after rich foods or a heavy drinking session. If you suffer from chronic fatigue, headaches, allergies, candidiasis, high-blood pressure, PMS, hypoglycaemia, mood swings or menopausal problems the *Liver Detox Plan* could be the breakthrough you've been looking for.

Xandria explains clearly what the liver does and what can go wrong. By following a 4- or 8-week plan you can achieve greater vitality, energy and weight loss (if desired) and can repair the damage of your past lifestyle. The *Liver Detox Plan* includes meal plans, recipes and supplements that can dramatically improve your health and your life.